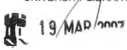

**Also available in the 'Current Issues in Midwifery' series:**

*Psychology for Midwives* by Ruth Paradice

*Health-related Fitness during Pregnancy* by Sylvia Baddeley

*Obstetric Litigation from A–Z* by Andrew Symon

*Demystifying Qualitative Research in Pregnancy and Childbirth* edited by Tina Lavender, Grace Edwards and Zarko Alfirevic

*Challenges to Midwives* edited by Yana Richens

*HIV and Midwifery Practice* by Jane Bott

*Birthing Positions* by Regina Coppen


Series editor: Jane Bott

# Perineal Care: An international issue

edited by

## Christine Henderson and Debra Bick

Quay Books
MA Healthcare Limited

Quay Books Division, MA Healthcare Limited, Jesses Farm, Snow Hill, Dinton, Salisbury,
Wiltshire SP3 5HN

British Library Cataloguing-in-Publication Data
A catalogue record is available for this book

© MA Healthcare Limited 2005
ISBN 1 85642 276 3

Printed in the UK by Cromwell Press, Trowbridge, Wiltshire

# Contents

# List of contributors

Debra Bick RM, BA (Hons), MMedSc, PhD is Professor of Midwifery and Women's Health, Centre for Research in Midwifery and Childbirth, Faculty of Health and Human Sciences, Thames Valley University, London, United Kingdom.

Christine Davies is completing a Bachelor of Arts degree and is a Research Assistant at the Ottawa Health Research Institute, Ottawa, Canada.

Cathryn Glazener MD, PhD, FRCOG is Senior Clinical Research Fellow in Health Services Research, University of Aberdeen, Scotland and Editor, Cochrane Incontinence Review Group.

Ian D Graham PhD is Associate Professor of Nursing, University of Ottawa and Senior Social Scientist and Associate Director of the Clinical Epidemiology Program, Ottawa Health Research Institute, Otawa, Canada.

Christine Henderson RM, RN, MA (Warwick), MTD, DPHE (Surrey), DipN (Lond) is Research Fellow at the School of Health Sciences, University of Birmingham, United Kingdom and editor of the *British Journal of Midwifery*.

Christine Kettle SRN, SCM, Dip Mid, PhD, is Clinical Midwife Specialist, Academic Unit of Obstetrics and Gynaecology, University Hospital of North Staffordshire, United Kingdom.

Alison Metcalfe PhD, BSc (Joint Hons), RN is Research Fellow, School of Health Sciences, University of Birmingham, United Kingdom.

Karen Rosen is Development Education Officer at Interact Worldwide, a human rights charity which works with local partner organizations in developing countries to provide sexual and reproductive health and rights services. Interact Worldwide, Studio 325, Highgate Studios, 53–79 Highgate Road, London NW5 1TL, online at: www.interactworldwide.org

Abdul Sultan MD, FRCOG is Consultant Obstetrician and Gynaecologist, Department of Obstetrics and Gynaecology, Mayday University Hospital, London, United Kingdom.

Ranee Thakar MD, MRCOG is Consultant Obstetrician and Urogynaecologist, Department of Obstetrics and Gynaecology, Mayday University Hospital, London, United Kingdom.

Susan Tohill PG Dip, BSc (Hons) Midwifery, RM, RN is Midwifery Researcher, Birmingham Heartlands and Solihull NHS Trust, Birmingham, United Kingdom.

# Foreword

The birth of a baby is far from the end of the process of having a baby. It is an important new beginning that brings with it many exciting changes and challenges for women and their partners. For thousands of women each year the start of life as a new family is complicated by the aftermath of perineal trauma. Women tell us how the quality of their lives is affected at this special time, and how difficult it is to try and establish breastfeeding and to enjoy time with their babies when the pain and discomfort of stitches makes it hard to find any position that is comfortable.

Many women have expressed surprise at the levels of pain and say how ill prepared they felt for the range of physical symptoms they experienced postnatally, and for the length of time some of these symptoms lasted. Sound, up-to-date information about their pelvic floor muscles, how the perineum responds during labour, and the nature of perineal trauma and its potential consequencs is vital antenatally if women are to avoid the shock that some of them clearly experience in relation to their perineum. During labour they value being able to work more closely in partnership with their midwife to avoid perineal trauma wherever possible.

*I would like to have been encouraged to breathe the baby out — I wasn't told to push but I did because I was excited. I think that if my midwife had encouraged me to let my body do the work I might not have torn.*

Postnatally, women tell us that they would like more awareness and sensitivity from health professionals regarding the pain and longer term psychological effects of perineal trauma.

I welcome this book as a most useful resource, bringing together and exploring as it does some of the most up-to-date research and information in this field. It will provide midwives, doctors, childbirth educators and expectant parents with that vital information that might lead to greater awareness, a reduction in perineal trauma and hopefully also highlight areas for further research.

Gillian Fletcher
National Childbirth Trust President
United Kingdom
August 2004

# Preface

The idea for this book evolved over several meetings with colleagues from the University of Birmingham to discuss the launch of the perineal tear assessment tool described in *Chapter 6*. The background to the development of the tool highlighted that practice to prevent, minimise and manage perineal trauma continued to persist uninformed by evidence of effectiveness, and with little opportunity for women to discuss how they could contribute to their care. It was also clear that limited attention was given to ensure that those caring for women in the immediate postpartum period were trained to identify accurately the extent of trauma sustained or, if suturing was required, to use methods and materials which could enhance postnatal recovery. As a consequence, hundreds of thousands of women who give birth each year in the UK and worldwide, continue to endure pain and associated morbidity which may have been prevented or minimised. Whilst this morbidity may not be life-threatening, the short and longer-term consequences of unidentified or inadequately repaired and managed perineal trauma can be significant for the woman, her infant and her family. With this as the background, we felt that a book which specifically focused on this neglected aspect of women's health was pertinent.

Each chapter has been written by authors expert in their field and recognised internationally as such. Chapters are included on the anatomy of the pelvic floor, the management of perineal trauma, episiotomy, prevention of perineal trauma, the development of a perineal tear assessment tool, health after childbirth, and postpartum care of the perineum. Some chapters present evidence for the first time. For example, the chapter on episiotomy includes latest data on episiotomy rates worldwide. A chapter specifically devoted to the issues faced by women who give birth in developing countries, such as obstetric fistula, is also included, highlighting the very real danger pregnancy and childbirth still present to millions of women in the twenty-first century. That maternal mortality and major morbidity continue to affect such huge numbers of women worldwide must be addressed if the lives of current and future generations of women and their families are to improve. We make no apologies for including this as our opening chapter.

Whilst the book covers all aspects of perineal care, it is possible to read each chapter in isolation. A quick reference guide is also included to enable readers more readily to find specific information of interest. We hope that you will find the book a valuable resource.

Christine Henderson, School of Health Sciences, University of Birmingham
Debra Bick, Centre for Research in Midwifery and Childbirth,
Thames Valley University, London
August 2004

# Introduction: guide to chapters

*Christine Henderson and Debra Bick*

## Chapter 1: Reproductive issues in less developed countries

*Karen Rosen*

❖ Pregnancy related complications are the leading causes of death and disability for women aged fifteen to forty-nine in developing countries.

❖ Maternal mortality represents the greatest disparity between rich and poor countries, with 99% of all maternal deaths occurring in the developing world.

❖ The major causes of maternal death worldwide are haemorrhage, sepsis, complications of unsafe abortions, eclampsia and prolonged or obstructed labour. Yet for each of these problems relatively simple and cheap preventative measures can be instigated.

❖ For each maternal death a further fifteen to thirty women suffer from debilitating injury, infection or illness in the form of anaemia, infertility, pelvic pain, incontinence or obstetric fistula.

❖ Two critical factors are essential if maternal mortality and morbidity are to be reduced in the developing world: the availability of a skilled attendant at all deliveries; and the availability of emergency obstetric care when complications arise.

❖ The above factors present a healthcare challenge especially when considering many women deliver in inaccessible rural areas. However, projects such as the Centre for Development Studies (CDS) project in Bangladesh offers a simple example of how local and effective measures can seriously reduce obstetric risk.

❖ Ensuring safe motherhood requires support from families, communities as well as governments and international organisations. However, when considered globally, the cost is relatively cheap, approximately three US dollars per person per year for a low income family.

# Chapter 2: Women's health after delivery

*Cathryn Glazener*

❖ Health problems of one kind or another occur in as many as seventeen in every twenty women following childbirth. These present as new health problems persisting for six weeks or more in about half the women.

❖ For the postnatal woman the most common morbidity in hospital after tiredness is a painful perineum.

❖ Perineal injury during childbirth results in perineal pain and dyspareunia.

❖ Both suturing and forceps delivery contribute to the severity of the pain.

❖ Assisted vaginal delivery and episiotomy double the risk of perineal pain, but there is evidence to suggest that more rest in hospital prior to transfer home halved it. This highlights the importance of reducing perineal injury and suggests that enhanced care postnatally is necessary.

❖ Interventions for prevention and treatment must be based on good quality evidence from randomised controlled trials.

# Chapter 3: Anatomy of the pelvic floor

*Christine Kettle*

❖ It is important for health professionals to understand and have a good working knowledge of the anatomy and function of the structures involved during the whole episode of childbirth.

❖ This knowledge is critical if trauma to the perineum is to be minimised.

❖ Knowledge of the distribution of the tissues and muscles damaged during birth is vital when repair of perineal trauma is performed to reduce morbidity.

❖ New technology has enabled visualisation of the exact nature and location of damage to the pelvic floor.

❖ Perineal trauma can be sub-divided into four classifications according to the extent of the tissue damage.

## Chapter 4: The management of perineal trauma

*Christine Kettle*

❖ Perineal injury has occurred during childbirth throughout the ages and various methods and materials have been used by accoucheurs in an attempt to restore the integrity of severely traumatised tissue. However, appropriate and effective management is a continuing problem.

❖ In the UK, midwives are responsible for suturing the majority of perineal trauma sustained following spontaneous vaginal delivery. There are wide variations in techniques and materials used for perineal repair. The rationale for the suturing method chosen often originates from the way the practitioner was first taught, or 'tradition', rather than clinical evidence.

❖ There is great diversity in practice in the way suturing of perineal trauma is taught, supervised, and assessed and there are no national or international guidelines relating to the training of operators.

❖ If practitioners are appropriately trained and assessed they are more likely to provide a high standard of repair which will directly effect the short- and long-term morbidity suffered by women following childbirth.

❖ Knowledge of the anatomy of the pelvic floor, wound and tissue healing is critical in managing perineal trauma and reducing morbidity.

❖ Current evidence suggests that perineal trauma should be repaired using the continuous non-locking technique to re-approximate all layers (vagina, perineal muscles and skin) with a more rapidly absorbing polyglactin 910 (Vicryl Rapide™ ) suture material.

## Chapter 5: Episiotomy: the unkindest cut that persists

*Ian D Graham and Christine Davies*

❖ Episiotomy is the surgical enlargement of the birth canal by an incision of the perineum at the time of birth. There are two types: midline and medio-lateral.

❖ The routine use of episiotomy was based on assumption of benefit rather than evidence of benefit.

❖ Current evidence arising from systematic reviews and randomised controlled trials demonstrates that the restrictive use of episiotomy does less harm than the routine use of episiotomy.

❖ There is widespread variation in the use of episiotomy indicating that its use is not evidence based. Episiotomy rates vary internationally with a very high incidence in Latin America, Eastern and Central Europe.

❖ The performance of the surgery often also varies within the same professional groups implying that it is not clinical factors that determine its use, but rather the beliefs and practice of the care giver.

❖ Many non-clinical factors also determine its use, including; the nature of childbirth, beliefs about women, and even race, class and ethnicity issues.

❖ The emphasis on customer-led care and client choice has influenced the use of episiotomy. Encouraging women to question their care and express preferences is a strategy that should be used to change professional behaviour.

❖ An important pre-condition for reducing the use of episiotomy will be to ensure the transfer of evidence about its use into the knowledge base of indigenous and local providers in all countries.

## Chapter 6: Perineal tear assessment and the development of the Peri-Rule™

*Susan Tohill and Alison Metcalfe*

❖ To date there is a lack of objective assessment and measurement of perineal trauma.

❖ Assessment of perineal trauma has rested mainly on midwives and doctors observing the trauma and classifying it in accordance with available guidance or using their own clinical judgement.

❖ The development of the Peri-Rule™ provides the first pragmatic tool for the measurement and assessment of perineal tears. The tool was developed for a study that examined outcomes of surturing or non-suturing of the perineum.

❖ The Peri-Rule™ was tested for its reliability by midwives across four maternity units in the United Kingdom.

❖ The Peri-Rule™ consists of a single use measuring device made of medical grade soft plastic with a millimetre scale rule and an assessment pro-forma.

❖ Midwives learnt to use the tool in training sessions that took from five to ten minutes in duration. A CD-ROM providing tuition on the use of the Peri-Rule™ has been developed. Midwives have welcomed its availability and have found it immensely helpful in determining the degree of trauma and subsequent need for suturing. Further details can be obtained online: www.peri-rule.bham.ac.uk

❖ Women participating in the study reported that the tool caused no additional discomfort.

## Chapter 7: Prevention of obstetric perineal trauma

*Ranee Thakar and Abdul Sultan*

❖ Prevention and minimisation of perineal trauma is critical for the well-being of the woman, baby and family. However, how this is achieved can be problematic.

❖ The three levels of preventative strategies are primary, secondary and tertiary.

❖ Primary prevention includes elective caesarean section. However, the procedure is associated with increased mortality and morbidity and does not always prevent damage to the pelvic floor.

❖ Secondary prevention includes delivery techniques and positioning, however, there is limited evidence to support these. Episiotomy is the most used surgical procedure in obstetrics but can in itself give rise to associated morbidity.

❖ Whilst perineal massage is not harmful it has only been demonstrated to be beneficial when carried out during the antenatal period.

❖ Tertiary preventative strategies involve following-up those women who have had repairs or are having related symptoms by an experienced team. Ideally, all women should have endosonography and manometry when trauma has occurred.

## Chapter 8: Postpartum management of the perineum

*Debra Bick*

❖ Perineal pain may result from bruising or oedema of the perineal tissues, a spontaneous tear or episiotomy. The impact of pain can affect a woman's physical and psychological health and well-being, and her relationships with her baby and family.

❖ Despite symptoms being experienced by hundreds of thousands of women worldwide, identification and management of perineal morbidity has not been a high priority within routine postnatal care.

❖ Recent studies have assessed the effectiveness of a range of interventions to relieve perineal pain. Whilst some provide effective short-term pain relief, little is known about longer-term benefits.

❖ There is limited information on the onset, incidence and prevalence of perineal wound infection.

❖ Further work is required to inform the short and longer-term management of women who sustain third or fourth degree perineal tears.

❖ Asking women about their experience of perineal symptoms and ensuring that individual health needs are met using best available evidence of effectiveness, should be an integral part of postpartum care.

# 1

## Reproductive issues in less developed countries

*Karen Rosen*

In the twenty-first century, maternal mortality and morbidity continue to be serious problems in the developing world. Although reproductive healthcare has improved significantly in the past forty years, pregnancy and childbirth remain the leading causes of death and disability among women between the ages of fifteen and forty-nine around the world. Every minute a woman dies from complications of pregnancy or childbirth-around 529,000 per year (World Health Organization [WHO], United nation's Children's Fund [UNICEF] and United Nations Fund for Population Activities [UNFPA], 2003). Maternal mortality represents the greatest disparity between rich and poor countries with 99% of these deaths in the developing world, particularly Africa and Asia. In addition, for each woman who dies it is estimated that another fifteen to thirty suffer debilitating injury, such as obstetric fistula.

Although not necessarily predictable, childbirth-related problems are preventable and treatable with proper care and resources. In the developed world, widespread access to skilled attendance at birth and emergency obstetric services has reduced maternal mortality and severe morbidity rates virtually to zero. Women rarely die in childbirth and the very serious problem of obstetric fistula has been eradicated. In contrast, in less developed countries approximately one half of women giving birth do not have medically trained assistance, and should complications occur, few will have access to emergency obstetric care. However, as the case study from Bangladesh will show, education, family, community and government support will make pregnancy and childbirth safer and enable women to receive the care that they require and deserve in the case of an emergency.

Maternal mortality is the 'death of a woman while pregnant or within forty-two days of the termination of the pregnancy, irrespective of the duration and the site of the pregnancy, from any cause related to or aggravated by the pregnancy or its management, but not from accidental or incidental causes' (WHO, 1992). The five major direct causes of maternal deaths worldwide are haemorrhage (25%), sepsis (15%), complications of unsafe abortion (13%), eclampsia (12%), and prolonged or obstructed labour (8%) (WHO, 1999). Yet, relatively simple measures exist which can prevent or treat such problems. Bleeding can be controlled with drugs and the uterus massaged to stimulate contractions. Infection can be prevented by hygienic delivery conditions and awareness and management of sexually transmitted infections during pregnancy. Death and disability from unsafe abortion can be prevented through access to family planning information and services, care after complications, and where abortion is legal, safe abortion care. Deaths from hypertension can be prevented through monitoring during pregnancy and treatment with anticonvulsant drugs. Prolonged or obstructed labour (discussed in detail below) often occurs when the baby's head cannot pass through the mother's pelvis. This is more common in young girls whose pelvises have not fully matured and in less developed countries where malnutrition often leads to smaller stature of women. Early marriage and sexual activity should be discouraged, good nutrition in childhood and adolescence promoted, and Caesarean sections available in emergency situations.

Indirect causes account for approximately 20% of maternal deaths. These are preexisting conditions that are exacerbated by pregnancy or its management such as anaemia, malaria and HIV/AIDS. Women must be made aware of these conditions and treated for them before becoming pregnant, and should receive antenatal care throughout pregnancy if possible.

The maternal mortality ratio (MMR), the risk of death a woman faces once becoming pregnant, is the number of maternal deaths during a given year per 100,000 live births during the same period. The world MMR is estimated to be 400 per 100,000 live births (WHO, UNICEF and UNFPA, 2003). A few shockingly high examples from around the world are: Sierra Leone — 1800 deaths per 100,000 live births; Afghanistan — 1,700 deaths per 100,000 live births; and Haiti — 1000 deaths per 100,000 live births (Population Action International [PAI], 2001). These can be compared with Japan — 18 deaths per 100,000 live births; USA — 12 deaths per 100,000 live births; and the UK — 9 deaths per 100,000 live births (PAI, 2001). Both global and country estimates are likely to be underestimates due to the difficulty of data collection.

The maternal mortality rate is the number of maternal deaths in a given period per 100,000 women of reproductive age during the same time period. Maternal mortality reflects the general health, social and economic status of women in society and their access to health care. Maternal deaths are a direct result of poor health, poor nutrition before and during pregnancy, inadequate care during pregnancy and delivery and unsafe abortion. Maternal deaths significantly impact on society as a whole because if a mother dies her baby is less likely to survive, the family suffers an economic loss and the extended family and community face an additional burden.

A woman's lifetime risk of maternal death is the probability that she will die from complications of pregnancy or childbirth during her reproductive life-span (defined as between ages fifteen and forty-nine). This takes into account both the probability of becoming pregnant and dying as a result of pregnancy. In this regard, vast differences in sexual and reproductive health and risks exist between rich and poor countries. In the developed world we have access to high quality health care, life saving drugs and surgical procedures when necessary, as well as high contraceptive use and low fertility. This all contributes to good reproductive health and a lifetime risk of 1 in 2125 (PAI, 2001). In less developed countries the picture is very different and women face a 1 in 65 risk of dying in pregnancy or childbirth (PAI, 2001). A lifetime risk of 1 in 100 or lower is considered high risk. An even starker contrast exists between Europe, where a woman's lifetime risk of dying from maternal causes is 1 in 1895, and Africa where it is 1 in 15 (PAI, 2001).

The Three Delays Model, developed by Deborah Maine *et al* (1997) at Columbia University School of Public Health, is a framework explaining the social factors for maternal death. The first delay is in deciding to seek care for an obstetric complication. In many cultures, women and/or their families may not recognise the signs of pregnancy-related complications, nor realise how serious they are or that they can be addressed through the formal healthcare system. This may occur due to late recognition of the problem, fear of hospitals, the costs associated with professional care or lack of an available decision maker. The second delay is in reaching the healthcare facility.

Surveys in a range of countries show that many women would like to deliver in a health facility but are unable to do so because of distance and lack of transport. The third delay is in receiving emergency obstetric care at the health facility. This may be due to lack of staff, facilities, supplies or medication.

It is important that women, community and family members are aware of the signs and symptoms of complications in pregnancy and childbirth and know how to act on them. They should develop plans for emergencies, such as transport to health facilities that can provide care and insurance schemes where necessary. Healthcare staff should be trained, facilities upgraded, and referral systems made stronger. In the absence of such changes women will continue to die needlessly.

## The importance of skilled attendance at birth

The international community has started to take the problem of maternal mortality seriously. In September 2000, the Millennium Development Goals (eight mutually reinforcing goals designed to eliminate poverty and encourage sustainable development) were adopted, which include a 75% reduction of the 1990 maternal mortality ratios by 2015, and identify the proportion of births attended by skilled personnel as an indicator for this goal.

The term skilled birth attendant refers exclusively to people with midwifery skills (usually a doctor, midwife or nurse) who have been trained to proficiency in the skills necessary to manage normal deliveries and diagnose, manage or refer obstetric complications (WHO, 1999). For example, a skilled birth attendant can provide active management of the third stage of labour, which will help avert many cases of postpartum haemorrhage. However, current numbers indicate that only 53% of women in developing countries deliver with the help of a skilled birth attendant and only 40% of women give birth in hospital or a health centre (WHO, 1999). Figures are much lower in some countries.

For social, cultural, financial or practical reasons, many women in developing countries, particularly in rural areas, have their babies at home, either alone, with a family member or with the assistance of a traditional birth attendant (TBA). TBAs often learn basic delivery skills from their mothers but are not medically trained. Therefore, they are not considered skilled birth attendants. Controversy exists regarding the value of training TBAs as delivering with their assistance has not been shown to reduce maternal mortality. This is because they are often unable to recognise and manage complications and refer women to appropriate emergency obstetric care. However, they can provide culturally appropriate health education, emotional support and a link with the formal healthcare system. In addition, equipping TBAs with simple delivery kits may prevent some infection-related deaths. It is vital that TBAs are trained to recognise delivery problems and, if needed, guide women to medical care.

One reason so few deliveries have a skilled birth attendant present is that training in midwifery is neglected in many countries. In these places, there simply are not enough skilled attendants to provide adequate care or their skills are outdated. In addition, professionals may prefer to be in urban areas and it is logistically difficult to reach women who live in rural areas and give birth at home. Incentives should be given to encourage those with medical training to work in outlying areas where the need is often greatest.

# The importance of emergency obstetric care

Access to emergency obstetric care (EmOC) is critical because 15% of all pregnancies will result in life-threatening complications requiring emergency medical intervention; and up to 40% of pregnancies (WHO, 1999) may require some form of special care. Such complications cannot be accurately predicted and most often cannot be prevented, but can be treated. Skilled birth attendants should be present during all deliveries because they have the knowledge to manage and refer complications when necessary. To function effectively, however, they need to be supported by systems which ensure adequate supplies and equipment as well as efficient and effective methods of communication, transport and referral.

The safe motherhood community agrees that there should be at least four basic emergency obstetric care facilities and one comprehensive facility for every 500,000 people. A basic facility should be able to; administer antibiotics, oxytocic drugs and anticonvulsants by injection or intravenously, perform manual removal of the placenta and manual vacuum aspiration of retained placental material, and perform an assisted vaginal delivery. A comprehensive facility should be able to perform these functions as well as caesarean sections and blood transfusions. Providing such care requires trained professional staff, a good logistics system for medical supplies, a functioning referral system and good supervision.

The countries which have been most successful in reducing the maternal mortality ratio, such as Sri Lanka and Egypt, have gradually shifted to professional attendance at birth, facility-based deliveries, expanded health facilities, trained midwives and the encouragement of family planning. However, poor countries may only achieve this with political will, high standards of education and community support.

Maternal morbidity, the serious illnesses and injuries that women suffer as a result of pregnancy, has long been neglected. Estimates indicate that for every woman who dies from pregnancy-related causes, up to thirty suffer debilitating injury, infection or disease such as anaemia, infertility, pelvic pain and incontinence. These problems affect up to twenty million women worldwide (UNFPA, 2003), the majority in developing countries. One of the most severe and devastating of these injuries is obstetric fistula.

Fistula occurs when a woman, normally young, has a long or obstructed labour and cannot get a caesarean section when needed. The obstruction occurs because the woman's pelvis is too small, the baby's head is too big, or the baby is badly positioned. During obstructed labour, the prolonged pressure of the baby's head against the mother's pelvis cuts off the blood supply to the soft tissues surrounding her bladder, rectum and vagina. The injured tissue necrotizes, leaving a hole, or fistula. If the hole is between the woman's vagina and bladder (vesicovaginal), she loses control of micturition, and if it is between her vagina and rectum (rectovaginal), she loses control of her bowels. The baby is almost always stillborn.

The World Health Organization estimates that more than 2 million girls and women suffer from obstetric fistula with an additional 50,000 to 100,000 new cases occurring every year (Murray and Lopez, 1998). These estimates are based on women seeking treatment so are likely to be low. Fistula is particularly prevalent in sub-Saharan Africa and South Asia where early marriage and childbearing before physiological development are widespread, poverty, malnutrition and general poor health are endemic, and traditional care and home birth common.

In Niger (in French speaking West Africa) a recent study on fistula conducted by the United Nations Population Fund (UNFPA, 2003) found the average age of marriage was fifteen, but it reported that in some areas girls married as young as nine. Early marriage leads to early sexual activity and pregnancy, particularly since only a very small percentage of women in Niger use contraception, and of that number, only a few use modern methods. With eight children per woman (Population Reference Bureau, 2003), Niger has the highest total fertility rate in the world and its population is expected to increase dramatically over the next fifty years. UNFPA's study revealed 36% of girls aged fifteen to nineteen have either been pregnant or have at least one child (UNFPA, 2003). These factors, together with a preference for home births, a lack of skilled attendance at birth and limited access to emergency obstetric services, make fistula highly prevalent in Niger.

In many parts of the world social and cultural factors prevent women from receiving appropriate and timely care before, during or after birth. This leads to high rates of maternal morbidity. In some societies men are expected to make all the decisions regarding health care. Many women receive no antenatal care and may be expected to give birth at home without medical assistance. Shame, fear of medical professionals, inability to access care due to cost or distance, or unwillingness on the part of the family decision maker all contribute to pregnancy-related deaths and disabilities. For example, in some Islamic and Hindu communities the practice of purdah keeps women hidden from men outside their own family. Women may not be allowed to leave the house or can only do so if accompanied by a husband or male relative. This often makes accessing health care extremely difficult and, consequently, women may endure prolonged labour. In some cultures prolonged labour is blamed on infidelity by the woman and she is expected to endure it as punishment.

Harmful traditional practices such as female genital mutilation (FGM) may place girls and women at increased risk for fistula and other childbirth-related problems. FGM constitutes all procedures which involve partial or total removal of the external female genitalia or injury to the female genital organs, whether for cultural or any other non-therapeutic reasons. It is estimated that over 100 million girls and women have undergone FGM and each year a further two million girls are at risk (WHO, 2000). In Niger, 22% of the women with fistula who received repairs in 2002 had also experienced some form of FGM (UNFPA, 2003).

There are several different types of FGM, the most extreme of which may be the gishiri cut practiced in Nigeria among the Hausa people. It is used to widen the vagina for consummation of an early marriage or to treat various gynaecological problems, often during pregnancy and childbirth. A cut is made with an unsterilised instrument in the anterior wall of the vagina. This can put women at risk for fistula if the blade ends up in the bladder or rectum. A study done in three hospitals in south west Nigeria examined the relationship between FGM and complications at delivery. When all pregnancies were analysed, circumcised women were at significantly higher risk of tearing and stillbirths (Larsen and Okonofua, 2002). The study found that the increased risk of obstetric complications may be due to the scarring of perineal tissues which increased the likelihood of tearing and risk of haemorrhage.

Fistulas commonly occur during a first vaginal delivery. In societies where childbearing is highly valued this can seriously impact a woman's future. Having lost a baby and smelling constantly of urine or faeces, women with fistulas are often rejected by their husbands, shunned by the community and blamed for their condition. Untreated fistulas may lead to foot drop (nerve damage to the legs), making it difficult or impossible to walk, and possibly to infection, kidney failure and death. Many women live alone with fistula for years and struggle to retain their dignity in the face of this debilitating injury.

It is important to note that obstetric fistula is preventable and is virtually unknown in the developed world due to a decline in early marriage and pregnancy, education for girls, family planning and improved obstetric care. Every woman needs to have access to safe, hygienic Caesarean sections in the case of prolonged or obstructed labour. To reduce maternal mortality and morbidity it has been proposed that at least 5% of deliveries should be by Caesarean section (UNICEF, 1997). However, in many countries, only 1 or 2% of women receive Caesarean sections when their labour become prolonged or obstructed.

The good news for women who sustan an obstetric fistula is that reconstructive surgery can repair the problem and has up to a 90% success rate. After successful treatment most women can resume full lives and have more children. The Addis Ababa Fistula Hospital in Ethiopia pioneered fistula repair surgery. Open since 1974, it has helped over 25,000 women and has become a major teaching institution for surgeons all over the developing world. Hospital records indicate that most patients come from the Amhara region, which — according to a survey by the National Committee on Traditional Practices of Ethiopia— has the highest number of early marriages in the country. The hospital works with women's groups in the provinces to alert communities to the dangers of early marriage, potential complications of childbirth, and the critical need for emergency obstetric care in the case of complications. The hospital also informs women in rural and outlying areas about the existence of fistula repair surgery.

Unfortunately, the vast majority of women with fistulas never obtain treatment because they are unaware it is available, it is too costly and/or they are located at too great a distance from a hospital which can assist them. The procedure normally costs between $100–$400, which is well out of reach for many women. Although the Addis Ababa Fistula Hospital offers free bed and surgery, most places do not. Even when money can be raised, few hospitals have the staff, facilities or proper training to repair fistulas; many doctors doing such work in Africa are expatriates. The world capacity to treat fistula is estimated at only several thousand fistula repair surgeries per year, far too few considering there are several hundred thousand fistula victims in Nigeria alone. Many more doctors and support staff in Africa and Asia need to be trained to perform fistula surgeries and incentives must be given to attract skilled personnel to the areas with the greatest need.

The example of an Emergency Obstetric Care Committee from Bangladesh demonstrates how, with family and community support, maternal mortality and morbidity can be greatly reduced. Bangladesh is in southern Asia between Myanmar and India. A large percentage of people in rural areas live in poverty and have poor housing and sanitation. Life expectancy for women is fifty-nine years (Population Reference Bureau, 2003). The total fertility rate at 3.3 children per woman (Population Action International [PAI], 2001) has declined significantly in the past twenty years. However, the maternal mortality ratio is 850 maternal deaths per 100,000 live births, 8% of births are attended by skilled personnel, 26% of pregnant woman receive antenatal care, 49% of women use contraception and 11.5 out of 100 teenage girls aged fifteen to nineteen give birth each year (PAI, 2001). Traditionally, women have had low social status and little independence. Although the government raised the legal age of marriage for girls from fourteen to eighteen and has encouraged women's participation in the labour force, female literacy remains low (around 30%) and social preferences for early marriage, large families and male offspring persist. Many women give birth at home unassisted or with the aid of a TBA. All of the above factors make Bangladesh a country of high reproductive risk.

The Center for Development Studies (CDS), a partner of Interact Worldwide, provides reproductive health services in thirty villages in the Bogra district in the northern region of Bangladesh. At their twenty-four satellite clinics, CDS holds antenatal counselling sessions focusing on nutrition, the physical process of pregnancy and tetanus injections. It is mainly women who attend these sessions because most of the men are working. There are also two trained midwives who perform antenatal and postnatal checkups and encourage the women to return to the clinic within forty-two days of giving birth. In addition, CDS trains TBAs and provides them with refresher courses and a kit containing a rubber sheet, a needle and a cutting instrument.

To combat the 'three delays', referred to earlier in relation to the model developed by Maine *et al* (1997) CDS has formed an Emergency Obstetric Care Committee in one of the villages. This group which meets monthly, consists of ten to twelve volunteers who are mainly women, but also a few men who are leaders of the village. Once the TBA identifies a pregnancy as high risk she will attempt to convince the woman and her family of the importance of giving birth at the central clinic. If unsuccessful, the TBA alerts the Committee who will put further pressure on the decision makers to avoid a home delivery. In emergency situations, the Committee members will often visit the home to convince family members of the necessity of taking the woman to hospital. Due to their status in the community they are often more persuasive than the TBAs.

At the monthly meetings, the Committee collects a small amount of money (the equivalent of five pence in UK currency) from each member which is put aside as an emergency fund for problem births. When a labour complication occurs the TBA immediately notifies the Committee who will summon the CDS van which is available twenty-four hours a day to transport women to the clinic. The entire process usually takes thirty minutes. The fund covers the immediate costs of transporting the mother to the clinic and the Committee asks the family for reimbursement. However, if the family are very poor they may repay the loan in instalments, or in some cases, not at all. The Committee is currently saving to buy a van for the village which will ensure sustainability of the project, and has also enlisted a group of blood donors in the community.

CDS has provided three case studies which illustrate the successful functioning of the Committee and when reading these, it is important that the context of care is considered. The first focuses on an eighteen-year-old who gave birth at home with the assistance of two TBAs. Although the baby was successfully delivered the placenta was not and the mother started to haemorrhage. At this point the TBAs wanted to take her to hospital but her husband and mother in law would not allow it. One of the TBAs informed the Committee and three members arrived at the house with two paramedics from CDS. The paramedics attempted, but failed to deliver the placenta. They tried to persuade the husband to take his wife to hospital, but he refused claming he could not afford it. The Committee members present agreed to lend him the money and assured him they would donate blood for his wife. At that point he let his wife go to hospital where the placenta was delivered and she was given a blood transfusion. After two days she returned home. Both husband and wife attended the following Committee meeting to express their gratitude for saving her life. The husband asked the Committee to consider including him as a member in the future.

The second example concerns a very poor married sixteen-year-old in her first pregnancy. She received antenatal care from a trained TBA. She had abdominal pain twelve days before her due date and a vaginal examination showed that her cervix was undilated. The TBA was unable to convince her family members to take her to hospital as they feared she would receive a caesarean section which they did not approve of. The TBA went to the Committee who came and asked the family members to move the woman to hospital, but again they refused. The young woman in labour requested to be taken to hospital, saying she had saved some money for this purpose, but her husband continued to object. The Committee members who were present immediately brought over the Chair of the Committee and, on his request, the husband finally agreed and drove his wife to hospital in his rickshaw van. The baby, born after an episiotomy, was underweight and required oxygen. The doctors explained that if treatment had been delayed any further, the baby would likely have been stillborn. After two days in hospital both mother and baby returned home and the husband expressed his gratitude to the Committee.

The third case involved a twenty-two-year-old well-to-do woman in her first pregnancy. The woman suffered from high blood pressure and oedema during the course of the pregnancy and was under the care of a trained TBA. During her pregnancy she was visited regularly by the TBA and Committee members and told to be prepared for a hospital delivery, which her husband did not approve of. The day before her due date she felt her baby was not kicking in the womb as usual, and upon visit to the clinic, learned she had developed a large amount of oedema in the previous month. She informed her husband and mother-in-law of this fact but no action was taken. She then alerted a Committee member who came to persuade the family to take her to hospital. Her mother-in-law then agreed but her husband did not. Meanwhile, she was experiencing a lot of pain. A Committee member then brought over a religious leader who was on the Committee. The husband listened to him and the woman was taken immediately to a private clinic. After examination by a doctor they were told that the baby had died in the womb, a caesarean section would be required for delivery, and without it the woman might die. The husband did not want this done but a female Committee member made him understand the necessity of the operation. As a consequence, the operation was performed and the woman survived.

These three examples which reflect care deemed as the most appropriate within the local context, show that if individuals, families and communities are aware of the risks that every pregnancy and delivery entails, and of the necessity of medical care in the case of life-threatening emergencies, that lives can be saved. Although this can often be difficult due to local social, cultural or economic barriers, the Emergency Obstetric Care Committee in rural Bangladesh proves that with education, information, organisation and tenacity, tailored to the needs of, and involving the local population, positive change can occur.

Sexual and reproductive healthcare information, education and services are crucial if we are to reduce maternal mortality and severe morbidity in the developing world.

Family planning information and contraception will reduce unwanted pregnancies and allow individuals to exercise their human right to choose the timing, spacing and size of their families. Policies should encourage later marriage and childbearing and expand educational and economic opportunities for girls and women. Since we know that every pregnancy and delivery faces risks, the single most effective way to reduce maternal death is to ensure that a health professional with the skills to conduct a safe, normal delivery and manage complications is present during labour, birth and the postpartum period. In addition, communications, referral and transportation systems must be upgraded and emergency obstetric care facilities available and adequately staffed and supplied.

Introducing and sustaining safe motherhood requires support from families and communities as well as governments and international organisations. Reducing maternal mortality and morbidity is not costly. The World Health Organization estimates a comprehensive safe motherhood programme, including antenatal care, normal delivery care, essential care for obstetric complications, neonatal care, postpartum family planning and management of sexually transmitted infections would cost just US $3.00 per person per year for a low income country. It is time we spent the small amount required to avert millions of avoidable pregnancy-related deaths and disabilities that still occur around the world today.

## References

Larsen U, Okonofua FE (2002) Female circumcision and obstetric complications. *Int J Obstet Gynecol* **77**: 255–65

Maine D, Azakalan MD, Ward VM, Kamara A (1997) *The Design and Evaluation of Maternal Mortality Programs*. Centre for Population and Family Health, Mailman School of Public Health, Columbia University

Murray C, Lopez A (1998) *Health Dimensions of Sex and Reproduction*. WHO, Geneva

Population Action International (2001) *A World of Difference: sexual and reproductive health and risks*. The PAI Report Card

Population Reference Bureau (2003) *2003 World Population Data Sheet*. Population Reference Bureau,

United Nations Fund for Population Activities (2003) *Maternal Mortality Update 2002, A Focus on Emergency Obstetric Care*. UNFPA,

United Nations Fund for Population Activities (2003) *Obstetric and Fistula Needs Assessment Report: Findings from nine African countries*. UNFPA,

World Health Organization (1992) *International Classification of Diseases*. 10th revision. WHO, Geneva

World Health Organization (1999) *Reduction of Maternal Mortality*. A joint WHO/ UNFPA/UNICEF/World Bank statement. WHO, Geneva

World Health Organization (2000) *Female Genital Mutilation. Fact Sheet No 341*. WHO, Geneva

World Health Organization, United Nations Children's Fund, United Nations Fund for Population Activities (2003) *Maternal Mortality in 2000*. Estimates developed by WHO, UNICEF, UNFPA, Geneva

World Health Organization, United Nations Fund for Population Activities, United Nations Children's Fund (1997) *Guidelines for the Monitoring and Use of Obstetric Services*. UNICEF, New York

# 2

## Women's health after delivery

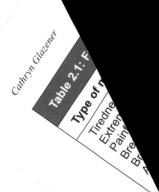

### Introduction

The postnatal period has been relatively neglected by health ‸
significant health problems for mothers have been largely unrecogniseᵤ.
clearly important to the mother, yet until recently, little was known about whaₜ
what problems arise and what help is available and effective. Both parents and ₙ
professionals traditionally regard it as a time to rest and regain health, but this is ofteₙ
not the reality.

### Postnatal health problems

Health problems of one kind or another occur in as many as seventeen in every twenty
women after delivery (Glazener *et al*, 1993; Glazener *et al*, 1995). These present as new
health problems persisting for six weeks or more in about half the women (MacArthur
*et al*, 1991). Although Caesarean section (CS) is known to result in increased maternal
morbidity (Hillan, 1992; Francome *et al*, 1993), it is less well recognised that women who
have an assisted vaginal delivery (AVD; forceps, breech or vacuum) report problems more
often (97%) than do women after a CS (89%) (Glazener *et al*, 1995). Although vacuum
delivery is preferable to forceps delivery for mothers (Johanson and Menon, 1999), the
babies suffer an increase in neonatal cephalhaematoma and retinal haemorrhages.

What are these health problems? The medical model of childbirth recognises
traditional complications such as anaemia, incontinence, depression, postpartum
haemorrhage, high blood pressure, puerperal sepsis, urinary tract infections and
thrombosis. Only the first three are common, however, (see *Table 2.1*) whereas the
rest, which pose a more serious risk to health, occur less often. Nevertheless, it
should be remembered that mothers still die from these complications. The latest UK
Report on Confidential Enquiries into Maternal Deaths (Confidential Enquiries into
Maternal Deaths Secretariat, 2001) found evidence of sub-standard care in 60% of
deaths, and were critical of the lack of agreed protocols for postnatal management. It
drew particular attention to unsuspected deep vein thrombosis (DVT) or pulmonary
embolism presenting as chest or leg symptoms in the puerperium.

What, then, are the more common problems? Women report tiredness, painful
perineum, anaemia, backache, constipation, piles, depression, headaches and incontinence
(*Table 2.1*), most of which are regarded both by them and health professionals as only
to be expected. Nevertheless, these add up to a considerable burden of ill health. This is
at a time when women are expected to look after not only themselves but also the baby,
and usually to resume full household responsibilities as quickly as possible.

| Morbidity | Range found in literature |
|---|---|
| ...ss | 36 to 89% |
| ...e tiredness | 12% |
| ...ul perineum | 22 to 49% |
| ...ast problems (breast feeding) | 33 to 45% |
| ...east problems (bottle feeding) | 18 to 28% |
| ...naemia | 23 to 47% |
| Constipation | 19 to 22% |
| Piles | 17 to 23% |
| Backache | 14 to 46% |
| Headache | 14 to 58% |
| Vaginal discharge | 12 to 16% |
| Urinary incontinence | 6 to 32% |
| Depression | 9 to 21% |
| Puerperal sepsis | 5 to 17% |
| High blood pressure | 2 to 9% |
| Difficulty vomiting | 5% |
| Abnormal bleeding/postpartum haemorrhage | 5 to 10% |
| Urinary tract infection | 3 to 8% |
| Wound infection (perineal) | 2 to 6% |
| Wound infection (abdominal) | 1 to 10% |
| Varicose veins | 1 to 8% |
| Dental problems | 3% |
| Thrombosis | <1% |

Data derived from a variety of sources in the literature. References available from author

In the past, women were protected from this pressure by a tradition of support, epitomised by the 'lying-in period'. More recently, the extended family and friends would still rally round to help. However, in these days of the nuclear family, and despite the theoretical entitlement to paternity leave, up to 20% of women report that they have insufficient help at home, even a year after delivery. The quality of postnatal care (PNC) also declines after the first two months (Glazener et al, 1993).

In response to the perceived lack of research in the field, the decline in quality noted by others (Filshie et al, 1981) and the decrease in length of postnatal hospital stay dictated by diminishing resources, I undertook a large, comprehensive survey of postnatal care in the 1990s (Glazener, 1999). The remainder of this chapter presents specific findings from that research, focusing on issues related to the perineum.

## Treatment of maternal morbidity

In a comprehensive survey, mothers were asked about their postnatal health at three time periods after delivery (Glazener et al, 1993). Of the 85% of mothers who reported at least one health problem in hospital, 85% received help or treatment for it (Glazener et al, 1995). Although just as many had problems on discharge home (87%), a smaller proportion (only two thirds) were treated, and of the 75% who had a health problem after the first two months, just over half received treatment (Table 2.2).

| Table 2.2: Number of women with any morbidity in hospital and proportion of health problems treated | | |
|---|---|---|
| **At least one health problem** | **Per cent of women** | **Per cent of women's problems treated or helped** |
| In hospital (n=1061/1249) | 85% | 85% |
| At home in the first two months (n=971/1116) | 87% | 69% |
| At home between 2 and 18 months (n=333/438) | 75% | 54% |

The pattern of decreasing help might be due to natural resolution of the problem or decrease in severity with time, but might also reflect a lack of recognition of the impact of continuing maternal morbidity by health professionals and mothers themselves.

## Perineal injury and pain

The best example of a health problem directly related to delivery, decreasing with time as the tissues heal and amenable to treatment is painful perineum. This mostly occurs after vaginal delivery. It is related to the method of delivery, the nature and extent of perineal injury and whether this was stitched.

In the PNC survey (Glazener, 1999), the relationship between method of delivery and perineal injury was as given in *Table 2.3*. Clearly, the majority of women who had an assisted delivery had an episiotomy, and most of the remainder had a tear. Interestingly, less than a quarter of women (22%) had no perineal injury at all, even if they had a normal delivery. Therefore the majority of women who deliver vaginally will need specialised care: this book summarises the current state of the science and art of delivering that care.

| Table 2.3: Perineal injury by method of delivery | | | | | | | | |
|---|---|---|---|---|---|---|---|---|
| Method of delivery | | Episiotomy | | Laceration | | Intact | | |
| | Total | No | % | No | % | No | % | |
| SVD | 896 | 168 | 19 | 463 | 52 | 265 | 22 | |
| AVD* | 172 | 152 | 88 | 9 | 5 | 11 | 6 | |
| Total | 1068 | 320 | 30 | 472 | 44 | 276 | 26 | |

* AVD includes forceps, vacuum delivery and vaginal breech

One significant consequence of perineal injury is failure to heal or wound breakdown. Of those who had a vaginal delivery (SVD and AVD combined) and were stitched, 17/707 (2%) reported stitch breakdown in hospital, and a further 19/622 (3%) at home, giving 5.5% in all who had significant perineal breakdown.

Wounds which fail to heal by primary intention may be resutured at once, or left to heal by secondary intention, or resutured after treatment of infection, with or without antibiotic cover. The one existing trial of immediate resuturing plus antibiotic cover compared with wound cleansing plus expectant care was inconclusive but suggested that serious consideration should be given to primary resuturing (with antibiotic cover) following rupture of perineal trauma during the puerperium (Monberg and Hammen, 1987; Johanson, 1995).

However, although wound breakdown is of importance, a much higher proportion of women reported perineal pain.

## Painful perineum

The most common morbidity in hospital after tiredness was painful perineum (phrased in the survey of postnatal care in lay terms as 'painful tail end') (Glazener *et al*, 1995; Glazener, 1999). In hospital, 42% of women reported this problem, of whom 79% were treated. This resolved rapidly at home (22% had pain, of whom 48% were treated), falling to 10% with pain after two months, of whom 44% received help. The fall in prevalence was significant both at two months and subsequently (P<0.001). Surprisingly, 6% of women reported new perineal pain first arising after they had gone home from hospital, and a further 2% subsequently (*Table 2.4*), but the overall trend was for resolution with time.

| Table 2.4: Incidence of perineal pain after childbirth | | | | | | | | |
|---|---|---|---|---|---|---|---|---|
| Painful perineum | In hospital | At home before 2 months | | | | At home between 2 and 18 months | | |
| | | Overall | Persisting | New | P value | Overall | Persisting | New | P value |
| | 525 | 249 | 208 | 41 | <0.001 | 43 | 38 | 5 | <0.001 |
| Total (N) | (1249) | (1116) | (469) | (647) | | (438) | (192) | (246) | |
| Per cent | 42% | 22% | 44% | 6% | | 10% | 20% | 2% | |

P value refers to comparison between hospital and before two months, and before two months and two to eighteen months, (ie. adjoining periods) by McNemar test

The overall figures disguise the differential effect of mode of delivery. Perineal pain was significantly related to method of delivery at each time point: clearly, assisted vaginal delivery was most commonly associated with the pain (*Table 2.5*), due to the high rate of episiotomy (88%, *Table 2.3*) and stitching (99%, *Table 2.5*). In contrast, only 70% of women were stitched after an SVD. Interestingly, a few women delivered by CS reported perineal pain, showing that perineal discomfort could be due to other pathologies. The most striking finding, however, was the long-term persistence of perineal pain (30%) after assisted vaginal delivery (*Table 2.5*).

## Table 2.5: Perineal pain by method of delivery

| Method of delivery | Number | Number with pain | Per cent | P-value* |
|---|---|---|---|---|
| **In hospital** | | | | |
| SVD | 896 | 372 | 42 | |
| AVD** | 172 | 144 | 84 | <0.001 |
| CS | 181 | 9 | 5 | |
| **At 2 months** | | | | |
| SVD | 806 | 155 | 19 | |
| AVD** | 149 | 88 | 59 | <0.001 |
| CS | 161 | 6 | 4 | |
| **At 12–18 months** | | | | |
| SVD | 310 | 23 | 7 | |
| AVD** | 63 | 19 | 30 | <0.001 |
| CS | 65 | 1 | 2 | |

* Chi squared test
** AVD includes forceps, vacuum delivery and vaginal breech

In order to identify factors which might be amenable to treatment, a logistic regression analysis was carried out to pick out which were the most important preceding factors associated with perineal pain. This analysis selected, in order of statistical importance:

- having any perineal stitches (rather than only for an episiotomy)
- being primiparous
- having an assisted vaginal delivery
- using entonox for analgesia in labour.

Notably, it was the use of stitches rather than whether these were for an episiotomy or tear that was the most important factor. Although these four factors are inter-related (primiparous women are more likely to have stitches, an assisted vaginal delivery and use entonox), nevertheless each contributed extra risk for having a painful perineum. (Women were also less likely to have perineal pain if they had an emergency CS or if they did not live with a partner, but the latter would not be amenable to intervention and increasing the Caesarean section rate simply to reduce perineal pain is not advisable.)

This analysis would therefore suggest that avoiding the need for stitching and reducing the assisted vaginal delivery rate might reduce perineal pain. Secondly, although not tested here, improving methods of management of the stitched perineum might reduce the impact of the pain.

Of women who had perineal pain in hospital, 44% continued to report it at home at first (*Table 2.4*, persisting pain). The prolonged effect of forceps delivery on perineal pain has been noted by others (Johanson *et al*, 1993a; Brown and Lumley, 1998). Assisted vaginal delivery and episiotomy both doubled the risk, but more rest in hospital halved it. Again, this highlights the importance of reducing perineal injury, and suggests that enhanced postnatal care (eg. more rest) may be helpful.

Only 6% of women reported painful perineum at home at two months if they had not experienced it previously in hospital (*Table 2.4*, new symptom). Episiotomy and a longer stage two in labour predicted it, as did a shorter stay in hospital. These were, therefore, women who were discharged home quickly despite an episiotomy and a long second stage: midwives should increase their level of vigilance in these circumstances.

Of those women who reported it in hospital or at home, 20% continued to experience it beyond two months (*Table 2.4*). A further 2% reported subsequent new perineal pain (*Table 2.4*), but there was not enough information to suggest why this occurred.

## Effect on intercourse

Problems with difficult or painful intercourse were also significantly related to perineal pain (Glazener, 1997): of 237 women who had perineal pain at two months, 51% had pain or difficulty with intercourse, vs 22% of 838 women with no pain (P<0.001); and 52% of 42 women vs 16% of 388 thereafter (P<0.001), suggesting a clear causal association. This confirms Johanson's report of 69% with perineal pain having short-term dyspareunia compared with 22% who did not have perineal pain, and 36% vs 16% having dyspareunia at one year (Johanson *et al*, 1993b).

## Long-term effects

The relationship between perineal injury, perineal pain and dyspareunia suggests that there may be a long-term effect on maternal well-being which might be expected to have implications for the marital relationship and perhaps the future stability of the family unit. Avoidance or minimisation of injury, and attention to good perineal care might have far-reaching benefits for mothers. Randomised controlled trials of alternative approaches to obstetric management and perineal care should include dyspareunia as an outcome measure.

Paternal leave, better postnatal support and more vigilance from health professionals might help to reduce the burden of maternal morbidity. This should improve the health of not only the mother, but also the baby and the whole family unit, but any new interventions should be tested by randomised controlled trial before wholesale adoption.

## Acknowledgements

*Dr C Glazener was supported by a Wellcome Trust Training Fellowship in Health Services Research, and a supplementary grant from the Grampian Regional Health Board Research Commitee. The Health Services Research Unit is funded by the Chief Scientist Office of the Scottish Executive Health Department, but the views expressed in this chapter are those of the author, not the funding bodies.*

# References

Brown S, Lumley J (1998) Maternal health after childbirth: results of an Australian population based survey. *Br J Obstet Gynaecol* **105**: 156–61

Confidential Enquiries into Maternal Deaths Secretariat (2001) Why mothers die 1997–1999: the fifth report of the confidential enquiries into maternal deaths in the United Kingdom. Royal College of Obstetricians and Gynaecologists, London

Filshie S, Williams J, Osbourn M, Senior OE, Symonds EM, Backett EM (1981) Postnatal care in hospital — time for change. *Int J Nurs* **18**: 89–95

Francome C, Savage W, Churchill H, Lewison H (1993) *Caesarean Birth in Britain*. Middlesex University Press, London

Glazener CMA (1997) Sexual function after childbirth: women's experiences, persistent morbidity and lack of professional recognition. *Br J Obstet Gynaecol* **104**: 330–35

Glazener CMA (1999) Investigation of Postnatal Experience and Care in Grampian (PhD Thesis). University of Aberdeen

Glazener CMA, Abdalla MI, Russell IT, Templeton AA (1993) Postnatal care: a survey of patients' experiences. *Br J Midwif* **1**: 67–74

Glazener CMA, Abdalla MI, Stroud P, Naji SA, Templeton AA, Russell IT (1995) Postnatal maternal morbidity: extent, causes, prevention and treatment. *Br J Obstet Gynaecol* **102**: 282–87

Hillan EM (1992) Short-term morbidity associated with caesarean section. *J Clin Nurs* **1**:107–8

Johanson RB (1995) Primary resuturing vs expectancy for ruptured episiotomy. In: Keirse MJNC, Renfrew MJ, Neilson JP, Crowther C, eds. *Pregnancy and Childbirth Module*. 2nd edn. Update Software, Oxford

Johanson RB, MenonVJ (1999) Vacuum extraction versus forceps for assisted vaginal delivery. The Cochrane Database of Systematic Reviews 1999, Issue 2. Art. No: CD000224. DOI: 10.1002/14651858.CD000224.

Johanson RB, Rice C, Doyle M, Arthur J, Anyanwu L, Ibrahim J *et al* (1993a) A randomised prospective study comparing the new vacuum extractor policy with forceps delivery. *Br J Obstet Gynaecol* **100**: 524–30

Johanson RB, Wilkinson P, Bastible A, Ryan S, Murphy H, O'Brien S (1993b) Health after childbirth: a comparison of normal and assisted vaginal delivery. *Midwifery* **9**: 161–68

MacArthur C, Lewis M, Knox EG (1991) *Health after Childbirth*. HMSO, London

Monberg J, Hammen S (1987) Ruptured episiotomia resutured primarily. *Acta Obstet Gynecol Scand* **66**: 163–4

# 3

## Anatomy of the pelvic floor

*Christine Kettle*

### Introduction

The anatomy of the female pelvic floor is complex but, nevertheless, it is extremely important that health professionals have a sound understanding of the structures involved both during the process of childbirth and when undertaking repair of perineal trauma in order to minimise morbidity. The following chapter gives a simple overview of the bony pelvis and pelvic floor muscles, providing a baseline which can be explored in more detail if the reader wishes.

### The bony pelvis

The bony pelvis protects the pelvic organs and forms a framework for the attachment of the internal support structures, which holds the viscera in place. It is made up of the sacrum and coccyx posteriorly, the two innominate bones (ilium and ischium) anterio-laterally and the symphysis pubis anteriorly. The pelvis can be subdivided into the 'true' and 'false' pelvis. The true pelvis lies below the pelvic brim and contains the urinary bladder, uterus, vagina, fallopian tubes, ovaries, rectum and anal canal. The false pelvis is formed by the wide blades of the ilium and is situated above the pelvic brim. The boundaries of the outlet of the pelvis consist of the arcuate pubic ligament and pubic arch anteriorly, the sacrum and coccyx posteriorly, the ischial tuberosities and the sacrotuberous ligaments laterally.

Anatomically, the perineum extends anteriorly from the pubic arch to the coccyx posteriorly and it is divided into the anterior urogenital and posterior anal triangles. A line drawn between the ischial tuberosities divides the diamond shaped perineum into the anterior urogenital and posterior anal triangles (*Figure 3.1*). The anterior region contains the external urogenital organs and the posterior region contains the anal canal and sphincters (external and internal).

The perfect obstetric pelvis has an oval brim with an anteroposterior diameter (obstetric conjugate) of approximately 11cms (measured from the upper inner border of the symphysis pubis to the sacral promontory) and a transverse diameter of 13cms (taken between the two furthest points of iliopectineal lines). The smooth concave curve of the sacrum makes the shallow circular cavity of the pelvis spacious, the diameter of which is approximately 12cms anteroposteriorly and 12cms transverse (measurements taken through the plane of the cavity). The ischial spines are palpable on vaginal examination and are used as landmarks to assess descent of the fetal head, ideally they should not be too prominent. The obstetric outlet is described as diamond shaped with a transverse diameter of 11cms (measured between the two ischial spines) and an antero posterior diameter of 13cms (measured from the lower border of the symphysis pubis to the sacrococcygeal joint) (Stables, 2000). The pelvic diameters will vary slightly according to ethnic origin and individual build. Another consideration is that the pelvic shape can be somewhat deformed through the effects of childhood rickets or adult osteomalacia leading to difficult childbirth and extensive perineal trauma. However, this is very uncommon in developed countries through improved diet and lifestyle (Llewellyn-Jones, 1990).

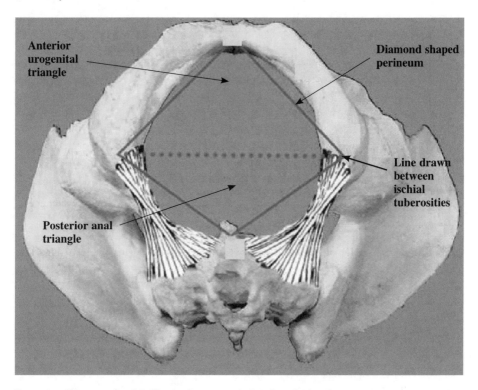

**Figure 3.1: Diagram of pelvis illustrating urogenital and anal triangle**

## Anatomical structures of the pelvic floor

The pelvic floor is formed by soft tissue that fills the bony pelvic outlet and forms a 'sling', which is higher posteriorly (Verralls, 1993). It extends from the pelvic peritoneum above to the skin of the vulva, perineum and buttocks below. The perineum can be subdivided into the anterior urogenital and posterior anal triangle (*p. 20*). In the female the urethra, vagina and rectum pass through its structures (*Figure 3.2*).

It consists of the following layers of tissue from the outside to within the pelvic cavity:

- skin
- subcutaneous fat
- superficial perineal muscles and triangular ligament

- superficial and deep fascia and ischiorectal fossae
- deep perineal muscles (levator ani)
- visceral layer of the pelvic fascia which thicken to form the supporting ligaments of the pelvic organs
- pelvic peritoneum.

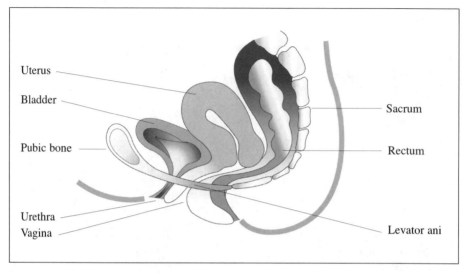

**Figure 3.2: Sagittal section of the female pelvis illustrating bladder, vagina and rectum in relation to levator ani**

In order to understand the structure of the pelvic floor, we will start by removing the skin, subcutaneous fat and superficial fascia of the external genitalia to reveal the underlying anatomy (*Figure 3.3*).

## Urogenital triangle

### The triangular ligament

The triangular ligament, which is also referred to by anatomists as the inferior fascia of the urogenital diaphragm, is formed by musculo-membranous tissue that stretches across the anterior portion of the pelvic outlet (Moffat, 1993). It is inserted into the urogenital triangle with the apex behind the symphysis pubis and the rami of the pubis and ischium forming the lateral borders. It fills the triangular space between the superficial perineal muscles (ischiocavernosus, bulbocavernosus and transverse perinei) and helps to maintain the normal position of the urethra and vagina (Burnett, 1969).

The urogenital diaphragm is composed of the inferior and superior facial layers with the deep perineal muscles, membranous sphincter of the urethra and pudendal vessels and nerves sandwiched between the fascia.

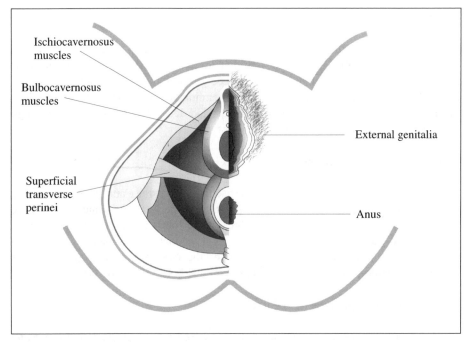

Ischiocavernosus muscles

Bulbocavernosus muscles

External genitalia

Superficial transverse perinei

Anus

**Figure 3.3: External genitalia with superficial tissue removed to reveal underlying superficial perineal muscles**

## Superficial perineal muscles

These are formed by following three pairs of muscles:

- bulbocavernosus
- ischiocavernosus
- superficial transverse perinei.

### Bulbocavernosus (or bulbospongiosus) muscles

These arise from a central point in the perineal body, encircling the vagina and urethra, passing anteriorly to be inserted into the corpora cavernosa of the clitoris. Some fibres may merge with the superficial transverse perineal muscle and posteriorly with the external anal sphincter. The main function of the bulbocavernosus is to constrict the vaginal orifice. The anterior fibres are inserted into the corpora cavernosa clitoridis and contribute to the erection of the clitoris during sexual activity.

Beneath the bulbocavernosus muscle lie the vestibular bulbs anteriorly and the greater vestibular gland of Bartholin posteriorly. The Bartholin's gland is a pea-shaped structure and its duct opens at the introitus just external to the hymen and medial to the labia minora. The main function of these glands is to produce a secretion to keep the vulva moist and well lubricated (Burnett, 1969).

## Ischiocavernosus muscles

These are situated on the lateral boundary of the perineum and arise from the medial surface of ischial tuberosities and ischiopubic ramus. The ischiocavernosus pass upwards and inwards along the pubic arch to be inserted into the corpora cavernosa of the clitoris. Some fibres interweave with the membranous sphincter of the urethra. The main function is to compress the crus clitoridis and delay the return of blood through the veins to maintain engorgement of the clitoris.

## Superficial transverse perinei

These arise from the inner surface of the ischial tuberosities and pass transversely across to unite into the central tendinous point of the perineal body and join with the bulbocavernosus in front. Some of the fibres of the transverse perineal muscles pass posteriorly to interweave with the external anal sphincter. The main function is to provide additional support transversely to support the lower part of the vagina and to fix the central tendinous point of the perineum (perineal body) (Burnett, 1969).

## The membranous sphincter of the urethra

The fibres of the membranous sphincter arise from one pubic bone and pass above and below the urethra to the opposite pubic bone. Due to the fact that it does not encircle the urethra it is not considered to be a true sphincter; however, it is capable of contracting to occlude the lumen of the urethra (Burnett, 1969).

## Deep transverse perinei

These thin narrow muscles pass transversely from each ischiopubic ramus to converge midline in the perineal body. Some of the fibres are inserted into the vagina. The deep transverse perineal muscles contribute to the supportive role of the urogenital triangle and assist with stability of the perineal body.

## The perineal body

This is a fibro-muscular structure, which is situated between the lowest third of the vagina in front, the anal canal behind and the ischial tuberosities laterally. Midwives and obstetricians refer to this area as the 'perineum'. When viewed in the sagittal plane, the shape is triangular with the apex uppermost. Each side of the triangle is approximately 3.5cms in length with the base being formed by the perineal skin. The pubococcygeus, bulbocavernosus, superficial transverse perinei and external anal sphincter muscles interlace within the perineal body. Thus, the support of the pelvic structures relies on the integrity of the perineal body. The lower part of the perineal body where most of the superficial perineal muscles converge is known as the central point of the perineum.

The perineal body receives blood from the pudendal arteries and venous drainage is into the corresponding veins. Lymphatic drainage is into the inguinal and external iliac glands and the nerve supply is derived from the perineal branch of the pudendal nerve.

## The vagina

This is a fibromuscular tube extending from the vestibule backwards and upwards to the cervix. It is lined by epithelial tissue that lies in folds or rugae to facilitate distension during intercourse and childbirth. The vagina lies in close proximity with the base of the bladder and urethra anteriorly and the rectum and pouch of Douglas posteriorly (Dilly, 1995).

It has a very rich blood supply mainly from the uterine, internal iliac and internal pudendal arteries. Lymph drains from the upper two thirds of the vagina into the internal and external iliac lymph nodes and the lower third drains bilaterally into the superficial inguinal nodes. The nerve supply to the upper part of the vagina is autonomic from the pelvic plexus but the lower part has a sensory supply from the pudendal nerve (Dilly, 1995).

# Anal triangle

The superficial transverse perineal muscles are located above the anterior margin of the anal triangle. The sacrotuberous ligaments and margins of the gluteus maximus form the lateral borders and the coccyx posteriorly. This area contains the anal canal, anal sphincters (internal and external), ischiorectal fossae and anococcygeal body.

## External anal sphincter

The external anal sphincter is a teardrop shaped circle of voluntary dark striated muscle, which surrounds the lower two-thirds of the anal canal (*Figure 3.4*). It is attached to the coccyx posteriorly by some of its fibres and it is shorter anteriorly in the female (Sultan, 1994a). The deep external sphincter is inseparable from the puborectalis muscle posteriorly. It is subdivided into three parts (subcutaneous, superficial and deep), which are not easily defined during dissection. The deep part of the external anal sphincter, assisted by the puborectalis muscle draws the anal canal forward to maintain the ano-rectal angle, which plays an important role in the continence of faeces. The puborectalis and external anal sphincter must relax to let the rectum empty. The action of the external sphincter is unique in that it is always in a state of tonic contraction. Its main function is to maintain closure of the lumen of the anal canal and to prevent uncontrolled passage of faeces and flatus by sustaining voluntary contraction.

## Internal anal sphincter

The internal anal sphincter is a thickened continuation of the circular smooth muscle of the rectum and is approximately 3cms long and 5mm thick. It extends downwards to enclose the upper two-thirds of the anal canal and the lower margin is approximately 6mm from the orifice of the anus. Just below the lower margin of the internal sphincter, the subcutaneous part of the external sphincter surrounds the lower end of the anal canal (Moffat, 1993). The longitudinal muscle of the rectum separates the internal sphincter from the external anal sphincter (*Figure 3.4*). This involuntary muscle is much paler in colour than the external anal sphincter and is not easily defined on dissection. The external and internal anal sphincters together form the anorectal ring, a firm structure that is easily palpated by inserting a finger into the rectum (Moffat, 1993).

The action of this muscle is entirely involuntary and its main function is to assist the external sphincter to maintain closure of the anal opening and to prevent involuntary passage of faeces and flatus, which is very important when sleeping.

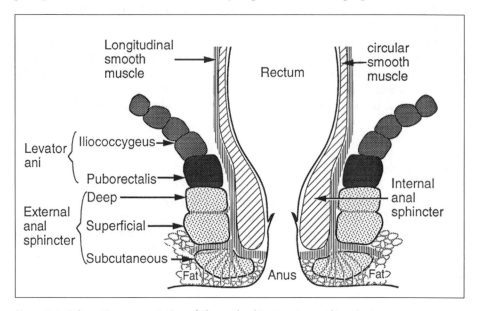

**Figure 3.4: Schematic representation of the anal sphincters (coronal section)**

### Ischiorectal fossae

The ischiorectal fossae are deep wedge-shaped areas. The parameters are formed by the external anal sphincter centrally, the lower part of the obturator internus muscle laterally, the levator ani muscles superiorly and the superficial fascia and skin inferiorly. It is important to understand that the fossa not only lies between the ischium and rectum but extends forwards to the back of the symphysis pubis (Moffat, 1993). The ischiorectal fossae are filled with fatty tissue and lined with deep fascia, including anal fascia and some of the obturator fascia, which lies below the origin of levator ani. The inferior haemorrhoidal vessels and nerves pass transversely across the space.

### Anococcygeal body

This is a fibromuscular structure that extends from the anus to the coccyx. Muscle fibres from the external anal sphincter and levator ani are inserted into the anococcygeal body. Its main function is to provide support for the anal canal.

### Blood supply

The arterial blood supply is from branches of the internal iliac and pudendal arteries and venous drainage is into the corresponding veins.

**Lymphatic drainage**

Lymphatic drainage is via the internal iliac glands.

**Nerve supply**

The nerve supply is from the perineal branch of the third and fourth sacral nerves, the inferior rectal and pudendal nerves.

# Deep muscles

The deep layer of the pelvic floor is approximately 3–5cms in depth and is principally formed from a group of muscles collectively known as the levator ani. Each levator ani muscle arises from the inner lateral pelvic wall, the posterior aspect of the pubis, the condensed fascia (the white line) that covers the obturator internus muscle and from the ischial spine to converge midline. From its broad origin, the levator ani muscle fibres sweep downwards, backwards and medially to be inserted into the upper vagina, perineal body, the anal canal, the anococcygeal body and the lateral border of the coccyx and lower part of the sacrum (Burnett, 1969; Llewellyn-Jones, 1990). The levator ani muscles form a strong 'sling' to support the pelvic organs and to counteract any increase in abdominal pressure when coughing or lifting which helps to maintain continence.

The levator ani is formed by the following muscles (*Figure 3.5*): pubococcygeus, puborectalis, iliococcygeus and ischiococcygeus.

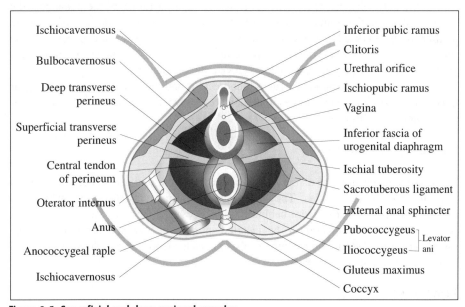

**Figure 3.5: Superficial and deep perineal muscles**

## Pubococcygeus

The pubococcygeus muscle is the most important part of the levator ani, both in size and function. It arises from the inner surface of the superior ramus of the pubic bones and from the anterior part of the obturator fascia and sweeps backwards to form U-shaped structures around the urethra, vagina and anorectal junction. The muscle fibres pass downwards and backwards below the bladder on either side of the urethra, upper vagina and anal canal posteriorly to be inserted in the anococcygeal body and coccyx. Some fibres terminate in the central tendinous point of the perineal body and others merge with the longitudinal muscle of the rectum. The main function of the pubococcygeus muscles is to provide support to the urethra, vagina and rectum. It also aids micturition and defaecation and constriction of the vagina during sexual intercourse.

## Puborectalis

The puborectalis muscle is the most medial portion of the levator ani muscle and marks the transition from rectum to anus. It arises from the lower part of the symphysis pubis and superior fascia of the urogenital diaphragm to converge with corresponding muscle fibres of the opposite side around the lower part of the rectum to form a strong sling. This helps to maintain the forward angulation of the anorectal junction, which plays an important part in maintaining continence of faeces.

## Iliococcygeus muscles

These are the lateral component of the levator ani and they arise from the tendinous arch of the pelvic fascia, which extends from the superior ramus of the pubis near the obturator canal to the ischial spines. The fibres sweep downward and inwards, joining midline to be inserted posteriorly into the anococcygeal body and coccyx. Some superficial fibres interweave with those of the external anal sphincter and transverse perineal muscles. These muscles help to elevate the pelvic floor.

When dissected the pubococcygeus, puborectalis and iliococcygeus muscles appear to be paler in colour, which suggest that they are fast twitch muscles and are capable of rapid contraction (Benson, 1992).

## Ischiococcygeus muscles

These are situated in front of the sacro-spinous ligament and are sometimes referred to as the coccygeus muscles. They are formed by triangular sheets of muscle and fibrous tissue, which arise from behind the iliococcygeus from the ischial spines and pass downwards and inwards to be inserted into the coccyx and lower part of the sacrum (Burnett, 1969). The function of these muscles is to stabilise the sacroiliac and sacrococcygeal joints of the pelvis.

## Blood supply

Blood is supplied from branches of the internal iliac and pudendal arteries and venous drainage is into corresponding veins.

## Lymph supply

Lymphatic drainage is into the inguinal and external internal iliac glands.

## Nerve supply

The nerve supply is from the third and fourth sacral nerves.

# Pelvic fascia

This connective tissue lines the pelvic walls (parietal fascia) and fills the spaces between the pelvic organs (visceral fascia). It extends from the pelvic peritoneum and abdominal muscles above to the levator ani muscles below and its main function is to provide support for the pelvic organs, whilst at the same time allowing them to distend during normal function.

## Parietal pelvic fascia

This is dense fascia that lines the bony pelvic walls and covers the surface of the pelvic muscles. Part of it thickens to form the white line of pelvic fascia, which gives origin to the levator ani muscles and thinner layers cover the piriformis muscle and pelvic diaphragm (superior fascia of the pelvic diaphragm). It extends below the levator ani to line the lateral walls of the ischiorectal fossa (Burnett, 1969).

## Visceral pelvic fascia

This consists of loose areolar connective tissue that fills the spaces between the pelvic organs and dense fascia, which encases the bladder, uterus, vagina and rectum. In areas where extra support is needed the fascia thickens to form supporting ligaments for the pelvic viscera. These ligaments contain condensed connective tissue and smooth muscle fibres, which have contractile and supporting functions (Burnett, 1969). The main supporting ligaments are:

- The transverse cervical ligaments (also known as cardinal or Mackenrodt's ligaments). These arise from the vaginal vault and supravaginal cervix and pass transversely in a fan-like way across the pelvic floor to be inserted in the white line of fascia on the lateral pelvic walls. These form the main supports of the uterus.
- The uterosacral ligaments. These arise from the supravaginal part of the cervix and pass backwards around the rectum to be attached to the front of the second sacral vertebrae. They support the uterus and maintain it in its normal anteverted (forward tilted) position.
- The round ligaments. These arise from just below the cornua of the uterus and pass through the inguinal canal and anterior abdominal wall to become inserted into each labium majora. They assist in keeping the uterus in its anteverted (forward tilted) anteflexed (bent on itself) position.

⌘ The pubocervical ligaments. These are fairly weak ligaments and they arise from the bladder base, vault of vagina and supravaginal cervix. They pass anteriorly to be attached to the inner part of the pubic bones and they provide support and stability for the bladder (Burnett, 1969; Verralls, 1993; Dilly, 1995).

## Main functions of the pelvic floor

The main function of the pelvic floor is to:

- support the pelvic organs, namely; the vagina, uterus, ovaries, bladder and rectum
- maintain intra-abdominal pressure during coughing, vomiting, sneezing and laughing
- aid defaecation and micturition
- facilitate childbirth
- maintain urinary and faecal continence.

## Pelvic floor dysfunction

During pregnancy the chorionic cytotrophoblast cells produce relaxin, which softens the pelvic muscles and ligaments allowing them to stretch to facilitate vaginal birth. After childbirth, the pelvic floor is able to resume its original supporting function in a surprisingly short time because of its remarkable elasticity. However, prolonged, repeated or extreme stretching, trauma or compression of the pelvic floor muscles and nerves may cause permanent damage resulting in loss of tone and elasticity. If the connective tissue and fascia, which supports the urethra and bladder neck is damaged during childbirth this may result in urinary incontinence due to ineffective transmission of intra-abdominal pressure (DeLancey, 1994; Zacharin, 1983).

More recent advances in magnetic resonance imaging have enabled professionals to visualise the exact nature and location of damage to pelvic supportive fascia and even assess when the levator muscles have been completely detached from internal pelvic walls (Kirschner-Hermanns et al, 1993; Tunn et al, 1998).

The introduction of anal endosonography and ano-rectal manometry has added a new dimension to evaluating the genesis of anal incontinence by allowing structural defects of the internal and external sphincters to be easily visualised. Prior to the introduction of endosonography it was hypothesized that anal incontinence was caused by damage to the pelvic and pudendal nerves during prolonged pushing which was associated with weakening of the pelvic floor structures and sphincters (Parks et al, 1977; Snooks et al, 1984). Pelvic floor neuropathy can be measured by electromyography, pudendal nerve conduction tests and assessment of pelvic floor strength using a perineometer (Allen et al, 1990).

Research carried out by Klein et al (1994) found that at three months postpartum, women who delivered vaginally with an intact perineum had stronger pelvic floor muscles compared to those with an episiotomy. This was assessed by performing electromyographic perineometry on the trial participants at thirty to thirty-four weeks gestation and at three months postpartum with a standardised perineometer. The study also found that incisions or lacerations to the perineal muscles were strongly associated with increased pelvic floor dysfunction. Therefore, it could be hypothesised that if perineal trauma is not repaired meticulously then the pelvic floor muscles may be weakened resulting in dysfunctions such as incontinence or prolapse. Unfortunately, there have been no randomised controlled trials of sufficient methodological quality to compare the effects of non-suturing of perineal trauma to suturing with respect to long-term pelvic floor muscle function (see *Chapter 4*).

Main causes of pelvic floor muscle weakness:

- pregnancy and vaginal birth including prolonged or difficult labour
- perineal trauma
- continual straining to empty bowels due to chronic constipation
- persistent heavy lifting
- chronic cough such as smoker's cough or chronic bronchitis and asthma
- obesity
- reduced oestrogen levels due to menopause
- lack of general fitness
- not carrying out regular pelvic floor muscle exercises.


# Perineal trauma


## Definition

Anterior perineal trauma is defined as injury to the labia, anterior vagina, urethra or clitoris. Trauma in this area is associated with less maternal morbidity. Posterior perineal trauma is defined as any injury to the posterior vaginal wall, perineal muscles or anal sphincters (external and internal) and may include disruption of the rectal mucosa.

Perineal trauma may occur either spontaneously during vaginal birth or the midwife or obstetrician intentionally makes a surgical incision (episiotomy) to increase the diameter of the vulval outlet and facilitate delivery.

## Classification and structures involved

Perineal trauma can be sub-divided into four classifications according to the extent of the tissue damage:

I.  *First degree*, which is very superficial and may involve:
    a. the skin and subcutaneous tissue of the anterior or posterior perineum
    b. vaginal epithelium
    c. a combination of the above resulting in multiple superficial lacerations.

II. *Second degree or episiotomy*, which is deeper and may involve:
    a. superficial perineal muscles (bulbocavernosus, transverse perineal)
    b. perineal body.
    This type of trauma usually extends downwards from the posterior and/or lateral

vaginal walls, through the hymenal remnants, towards the anal margin and it usually occurs in the weakest part of the stretched perineum. If the trauma is very deep the pubococcygeus muscle may be disrupted.

Less frequently the tear extends in a circular direction, behind the hymenal remnants, bilaterally upwards towards the clitoris causing the lower third of the vagina to detach from the underlying structures (Sultan *et al*, 1994a). This type of complex trauma causes vast disruption to the perineal body and muscles but the perineal skin may remain intact making it difficult to repair.

III.  **Third degree**, which is more severe and involves the superficial and/or deep perineal muscles and anal sphincter/s. More recently, Sultan (1999) and Keighley *et al* (2000) suggested that third degree tears should be sub-classified as:
a. 3a = less than 50% of the external anal sphincter damaged
b. 3b = more than 50% of the external anal sphincter damaged
c. 3c = including internal anal sphincter damage.

IV.  **Fourth degree tears**, which involve the same structures as above including disruption of the external anal sphincter and/or internal anal sphincter and the anorectal epithelium.

# References

Allen RE, Hosker G L, Smith AR, Warrell DW (1990) Pelvic floor damage and childbirth: a neurophysiological study. *Br J Obstet Gynaecol* **97**: 770–79

Benson JT (1992) *Female Pelvic Floor Disorders, Investigation and Management*. Norton Medical Books. WW Norton & Company, London

Burnett (1969) *The Anatomy and Physiology of Obstetrics*. Faber and Faber Limited, London

DeLancey JO (1994) Structural support of the urethra as it relates to stress urinary incontinence: the hammock hypothesis. *Am J Obstet Gynecol* **170**: 1713–23

Dilly (1995) Anatomy of the female pelvis. In: Turnbull's *Obstetrics*. 2nd edn. Churchill Livingstone, London

Keighley MRB, Radley S, Johanson R (2000) Consensus on prevention and management of post-obstetric bowel incontinence and third degree tear. *Clinical Risk* **6**: 231–7

Kirschner-Hermanns R, Wein B, Niehaus S, Schaefer W, Jaske G (1993) The contribution of magnetic resonance imaging of the pelvic floor to the understanding of urinary incontinence. *Br J Urol* **72** (7): 715–18

Klein MC, Gauthier RJ, Robbins JM, Kaczorowski J, Jorgensen SH, Franco ED *et al* (1994) Relationship of episiotomy to perineal trauma and morbidity, sexual dysfunction and pelvic floor relaxation. *Am J Obstet Gynecol* **71**: 591–8

Llewellyn-Jones D (1990) *Fundamentals of Obstetrics and Gynaecology*. 5th edn. Faber and Faber, London

Moffat DB (1993) *Lecture Notes on Anatomy*. Blackwell Scientific Publications, Oxford

Parks AG, Swash M, Urich H (1977) Sphincter denervation in anorectal incontinence and rectal prolapse. *Gut* **18**: 656–65

Snooks SJ, Setchell M, Swash M, Henry MM (1984) Injury to innervation of pelvic floor sphincter musculature in childbirth. *The Lancet* **2**(8402): 546–50

Stables D (2000) *Physiology in Childbearing*. Baillière Tindall, London

Sultan AH, Kamm MA, Bartram CI, Hudson CN (1994a) Perineal damage at delivery. *Contemp Rev Obstet Gynaecol* **6**: 8–24

Sultan AH (1999) Editorial: Obstetric perineal injury and anal incontinence. *Clinical Risk* **5**: 193–6

Tunn R, Paris S, Fischer W, Hamm B, Kuchinke J (1998) Static magnetic resonance imaging of the pelvic floor muscle morphology in women with stress urinary incontinence and pelvic prolapse. *Neurol Urodynamics* **17**(6): 579–89

Verralls S (1993) *Anatomy and Physiology Applied to Obstetrics*. 3rd edn. Churchill Livingstone, London

Zacharin RF (1983) Abdomino-perineal suspension in the management of recurrent stress incontinence of urine — a 15-year experience. *Obstet Gynaecol* **62**: 644–54

**4**

# The management of perineal trauma

*Christine Kettle*

## Introduction

Review of historical literature confirms that perineal injury has occurred during childbirth throughout the ages and that various methods and materials were used by accoucheurs in an attempt to restore the integrity of severely traumatised tissue. The earliest evidence of severe perineal injury sustained during childbirth exists in the mummy of Henhenit, a Nubian woman approximately twenty-two years of age, from the harem of King Mentuhotep II, of Egypt 2050 BC (Derry, 1935; Magdi, 1949; Graham, 1950).

It is interesting to note that most of the ancient writings on midwifery and obstetrics advocate the stitching of perineal trauma (Graham, 1950; Towler and Bramall, 1986). However, despite the fact that midwives were advised to stitch 'complete' perineal tears following childbirth, it would appear that this procedure was not routinely practiced. Eccles (1982) suggested that the reasons for not suturing might have been due to either 'resistance on the part of the patient or squeamishness on the part of the midwife'. One ancient midwifery book published by Thomas Raynalde in 1540 entitled *The Byrthe of Mankynde* recommended an alternative method of perineal repair, whereby pieces of linen cloth were stuck to each side of the perineal wound and then stitched together (Eccles, 1982; Rhodes, 1995).

Controversy regarding the best management of perineal trauma, relating to suturing following childbirth, continued throughout the centuries. Some accoucheurs believed

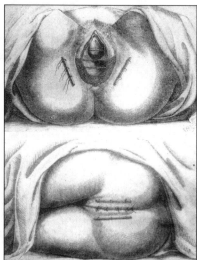

that it was much better to leave perineal trauma unsutured to facilitate 'ensuing' deliveries, whilst others argued that the outcome for women and their partners would be considerably improved if the trauma were sutured.

It was many years before perineal suturing became generally accepted. This may have been due to the fact that insertion of stitches would have been extremely painful for women because there were no local anaesthetics. Moreover, equipment was crude, aseptic techniques did not exist and most midwives were inexperienced in carrying out this procedure successfully. Indeed, up until the late nineteenth century, women with severe perineal damage were confined to bed for up to six weeks and nursed on their side with their legs tied together to encourage healing by secondary intention (Magdi, 1949).

**Figure 4.1: Perineal repair using wire sutures and lead strips**

## Formal midwifery training

Midwives throughout the centuries received very little formal training in the art and science of childbirth, until the late eighteenth century. Most of their skills relating to normal midwifery were passed down from mother to daughter. They were formally licensed to practice by the church during the sixteenth century and received some instructions from 'men-midwives' such as Willughby, Chamberlen and Smellie (Towler and Bramall, 1986).

In 1872 in the UK, the London Obstetrical Society set up its own Board of Examiners and issued certificates of competence to the many thousands of midwives who took the examination (Radcliffe, 1967). Following this, as a result of the 1902 Midwives Act, the Central Midwives Board (CMB) was established in England to regulate the training, supervision and registration of midwives.

## Training of midwives in perineal repair

In June 1967, midwives working in the UK were permitted by the Central Midwives Board (CMB) to perform episiotomies, but they were not allowed to suture perineal trauma (Myles, 1971; Silverton, 1993). Indeed, midwifery textbooks contained very little information relating to this particular area of childbirth. By June 1970 the Chairman of the CMB, issued a statement that midwives who were working in 'remote areas overseas' may be authorised by the doctor concerned to repair episiotomies, providing that they had been taught the technique and were judged to be competent, but the final responsibility rested with the doctor (Myles, 1971). However, it was not until 1983 that perineal repair was included in the midwifery curriculum in the UK when the European Community Midwives Directives came into force and the CMB issued the following statement:

> *Midwives may undertake repair of the perineum provided they have received instruction and are competent in this procedure.*
>
> (Central Midwives Board, 1983)

## Diversity of practice

Currently, in the UK, midwives are responsible for suturing the majority of perineal trauma sustained following spontaneous vaginal delivery. However, there are wide variations in both the techniques and materials used for perineal repair between individual practitioners and hospitals. The rationale for the suturing method chosen quite often originates from the way the practitioner was first taught, rather than being firmly based on clinical evidence. Indeed, a telephone survey carried out in 1995 revealed that out of twenty-one hospitals contacted within the West Midlands region of the UK, most were instructing midwives to undertake perineal repair using the interrupted technique with a diverse range of suture materials (Kettle, 1995, unpublished).

Greenshields and Hulme (1993) carried out a survey of women's experiences of perineal repair and recovery and midwives' practices in the UK and found that 81.4%

(n = 224) of the participating midwives used interrupted sutures; 14.2% (n = 39) of midwives used the subcuticular method and 4% (n = 11) used both techniques. Indeed, most were using outdated methods for perineal repair despite the overview of research by Grant (1989) which reported that women who had their perineum repaired with subcuticular sutures suffered less pain and required less analgesia than those repaired with transcutaneous interrupted sutures.

## Training deficiencies

Sultan *et al* (1995) carried out a survey in London, UK to assess trainee doctors' and qualified midwives' knowledge relating to perineal trauma and anatomy and to establish if they were satisfied with their training in this aspect of obstetrics. A random sample of midwives (n = 75) and doctors (n = 75), from neighbouring district general hospitals, were selected and asked to complete a questionnaire. The study found that only 20% of doctors and 48% of midwives considered their training to be of a 'good standard'. However, many of the answers relating to anatomy and classification of perineal repair given by these respondents were in fact incorrect. This research clearly highlighted the deficiency and dissatisfaction among trainee doctors and midwives with their training in perineal anatomy and repair, and recommended that more intense and focused training in this area should be provided. Similarly, consumers of midwifery services have also raised concerns and expressed dissatisfaction following their personal experiences of 'stitching', most of which were directly related to training issues such as the operator being 'inexperienced, unsupervised, having to learn by trial and error or just indifferent' (Rix, 1992; Brimacombe, 1995). Another important factor to consider, as stated by Lewis (1994) is that once the repair has been completed, most practitioners are unable to monitor the long-term effects of the procedure and have no means of auditing their own practice.

## Surgical skills training

It could be hypothesised that even if the best methods and materials are used for repair of perineal trauma, if the operator is unskilled or the procedure is not taught correctly then the outcome may be significantly affected. However, as stated by Mandel *et al* (2000), there appears to be little research evidence relating to the importance of acquiring and evaluating surgical skills, especially in obstetrics and gynaecology.

Recently, the media has highlighted some of the problems associated with poor training, bad surgical skills and variations in practice and outcomes between geographical areas (Dyer, 2001; Foster, 2002). With the initiation of clinical governance in the UK, hospitals and clinicians are now accountable 'for continually improving the quality of their service and safeguarding high standards of care, including dealing with poor professional performance' (Scally and Donaldson, 1998). However, there appear to be serious deficiencies and wide variations in the way practical skills are taught. As stated by Jelovsek (1995) most faculties teach 'factual knowledge very well', but residents are expected to 'arrive at the first operative experience having mastered some basics that no one was assigned to teach'. Similarly, student midwives have a detailed curriculum in the theory relating to perineal anatomy and repair but have very little opportunity to practice the procedure during their training. Most midwives do not become skilled in performing perineal repairs until after they are qualified. Furthermore, there are wide variations throughout the country in the way the procedure is taught, supervised and assessed, as currently there are no national guidelines relating to the training of operators.

The most common method employed to train healthcare providers in the 'skill' of perineal repair has been for the trainee to observe one or two, perform one or two under supervision and then perform the suturing unsupervised. The apparent limitations of this 'clinical' training lie in the time available for actually teaching the procedure. In addition, there may be limited opportunity to observe the procedure and there is no guarantee that a suitable patient scenario for a supervised session will occur within a reasonable time span after observing a perineal repair. Furthermore, it may take the trainee more time to perform the repair, causing the woman more discomfort and delay in physical contact with her baby.

Review of the literature found one small obstetric study (n = 11), which was carried out by Cain and Shirar (1996) to evaluate the effectiveness of using a three-dimensional model to teach repair of second-degree tears to family practice residents in Denver, USA. The researchers reported that eight months after the initial teaching session, 'learners were able to consistently perform the simulation and rated it to be superior to learning from textbooks'. They concluded that perineal repairs could be taught using a simple teaching model and that time spent supervising perineal repair in the delivery area might also be decreased. However, the findings of this study must be interpreted with caution, as there was no comparative control group. Further, well-designed controlled studies are needed to evaluate with certainty, the effectiveness and cost implications of using alternative methods of teaching repair of perineal trauma.

It is likely that practitioners who are appropriately trained and assessed will be more able to provide a consistent, high standard of perineal repair which might have a direct effect on short and long-term outcome in terms of reducing the extent of morbidity associated with this procedure; however, it is important that practice outcome are regularly evaluated.

## Management of perineal trauma

### Pathophysiology of wound and tissue healing

The process by which all wounds heal, including perineal trauma, is biologically complex and consists of several pathophysiological responses, including; coagulation, inflammation, matrix synthesis and deposition, angiogenesis, fibroplasia, epithelialization, contraction and remodelling. It is conventional to sub-classify these responses into three main phases, namely; inflammation, proliferation and maturation. However, these do not necessarily run in sequence but actually occur in parallel (Aljafri and Kingsnorth, 1998).

The inflammatory phase consists of a vascular and cellular response, which begins immediately after tissue injury and lasts between three to five days (Aljafri and Kingsnorth, 1998). The second proliferate phase occurs around three to four days and consists of granulation, wound contraction and epithelialization. This phase continues for up to three weeks (Tortora and Grabowski, 1993). Four to five days after injury, fibroblasts begin to produce large amounts of collagen, which is deposited in a random pattern with the interweaving fibres forming a source of intrinsic strength. The tensile strength of the wound continues to increase over the next few months, however it is able to cope with normal stresses within two to three weeks. The last phase is maturation or remodeling and this lasts for approximately three weeks to two years during which fibroblasts leave the wound and collagen is remodeled into a more organized matrix in response to the 'local stresses' (Aljafri and Kingsnorth, 1998). The collagen that produced the bulk of the wound gradually diminishes and the scar becomes quite dense due to loss of fluid and volume (Koopmann, 1995). The tensile strength increases with time but only reaches 70 to 80% of the original strength.

## Scar tissue

This differs from normal tissue in that the collagen fibers are arranged more densely. It also has fewer blood vessels and may not contain sensory neurons, hair or skin glands. The process of scar tissue formation is called fibrosis and sometimes it is so profuse that it is raised above the normal epidermal surface. If the scar tissue remains within the boundaries of the wound it is called a 'hypertrophic scar', but if it extends beyond into normal surrounding tissue it is called a 'keloid scar' (Tortora and Grabowski, 1993).

It is thought that the degree of scarring is related to the duration of time that the wound is allowed to remain in the inflammatory phase of healing. In addition, mechanical stress and tension along the suture line, especially when associated with excessive movement, will lead to a widened hypertrophic scar. The initial healing process may be enhanced by immobilization of the wound (Koopmann, 1995).

## Healing by primary or first intention

This is a simple process whereby wounds with closely adjoining edges and a small amount of tissue loss or damage heal fairly rapidly. For example, clean surgical wounds, episiotomies or perineal tears that have been carefully repaired will heal by primary intention with minimal scarring providing there are no adverse factors such as localised infection or haematoma formation. Epithelialization and contraction have a very small role to play in this type of healing (Koopmann, 1995).

## Healing by secondary intention

In contrast, when there has been a substantial loss of tissue or if, for example, a sutured perineal wound breaks down due to infection or imprecise approximation of the wound edges, healing has to take place by secondary intention. This is a more prolonged and complicated process whereby the defect is filled from the inner layer to the outward surface with granulation tissue containing myofibroblasts and capillary loops.

The process is assisted by wound contraction but if there is chronic delay in healing this allows the collagen fibres to mature and shorten, resulting in the pathological condition of wound contracture (Aljafri and Kingsnorth, 1998). This may cause tissue deformity and excessive scar formation with poor cosmetic results. Moreover, if the process is not supervised, or if the wound is neglected, there is an increased risk of localized infection spreading systemically which may be extremely debilitating. Occasionally, the granulation tissue is so prolific that it sometimes protrudes above the surface of the wound and it has to be cauterised otherwise the process of epithelialization will be prevented.

## Factors affecting healing

The rate and quality of wound healing and scar formation is affected by multiple factors, which can be categorized into local and systemic causes. Some of the local reasons for inadequate healing, include: persisting infection; a prolonged inflammatory phase due to the damaged tissue reacting to foreign materials such as sutures; inadequate blood supply causing hypoxia; haematoma formation; excessive movement; irradiation and locally applied drugs such as corticosteroids.

Perineal trauma following childbirth, which has been carefully sutured, generally heals very rapidly, usually within two weeks by primary intention. This is probably due to the fact that the perineal area immediately after parturition provides optimal conditions that are necessary for the promotion of quality healing. Some of these include increased vascularity, reduced exposure, moisture, warmth and a favourable pH of approximately 4.5 (acid) in which organisms are usually unable to grow (Quick and Thomas, 2000). Indeed, probably the most common local factor associated with delayed perineal wound healing and dehiscence is infection, which results in reduced collagen synthesis. This causes the wound edges to be softened and this may result in sutures 'cutting out' of the tissue with subsequent wound breakdown (Cuschieri *et al*, 2000).

The type of perineal trauma sustained may also have an effect on the rate and quality of healing. Three clinical studies found that there were more problems with early postpartum perineal healing associated with episiotomy as compared to spontaneous tears (Röckner *et al*, 1988; McGuinness *et al*, 1991; Larsson *et al*, 1991). They found that there was a significantly higher infection rate and that perineal wounds took longer to heal in the episiotomy groups. The question of whether an episiotomy incision should be mediolateral or midline is unclear (Carroli and Belizan, 2002). It is postulated that a midline episiotomy is easily repaired and is also associated with less blood loss, healing complications and pain than a mediolateral incision. However, it has an increased risk of extending and causing damage to the anal sphincter/s and rectal epithelium (Coats *et al*, 1980; Thacker and Banta, 1983; Klein *et al*, 1994).

Systemic factors, which impair the healing process are: hypovolaemia; malnutrition including protein, vitamin C and zinc deficiencies; excessive body fat; immune suppression; systemic steroids and metabolic diseases such as diabetes (Hogston, 2001). Age also has a direct affect on the rate of healing in that it proceeds more rapidly in the young providing that they are well nourished as compared to the older person who has a slower rate of tissue regeneration. In addition, cigarette smoking is thought to disrupt the pathophysiology of healing as it is associated with increased vasoconstriction of blood vessels and a reduction in oxygen to the wound site which may cause tissue ischemia and delay in tissue repair (Mikhailidis *et al*, 1983; Krueger and Rohrich, 2001).

A reduction in oestrogen levels in postmenopausal women is also associated with poor healing. Research carried out by Ashcroft *et al* (1997) demonstrated that systemic hormone replacement therapy (HRT) significantly improves the rate of cutaneous wound healing compared to age-matched controls not receiving HRT. Similarly, women who choose to breast-feed have low levels of oestrogen due to hyperprolactinaemia. However, there appear to be no research studies carried out specifically to investigate the effects of reduced oestrogen levels on the rate and quality of perineal wound healing during the early postpartum period.

## Non-suturing of perineal trauma

There are increasing numbers of midwives in the UK who are leaving perineal trauma unsutured without robust evidence to support this practice. To date, there have been three small retrospective studies carried out in the UK and two small randomised controlled trials carried out in Sweden and Scotland to evaluate the effects of leaving spontaneous perineal tears unsutured (defined as first and second degree trauma) (Head, 1993; Clement and Reed, 1999; Wood, 1999; Lundquist *et al*, 2000; Fleming *et al*, 2003).

Head (1993) sent questionnaires to seventy-five multiparous women who had experienced perineal sutures for at least one of their deliveries. Sixty-two were returned and seven women who reported never having stitches following childbirth were excluded from the study. Participants (n = 55) were asked to recall their experiences of perineal trauma following their deliveries in relation to pain, healing and infection and to compare injuries, which had been sutured to those that had been left unsutured. Head (1993) reported that the study showed a 'satisfactory outcome for women with perineal tears that were left unsutured' but the long-term effects were not known. The validity of the findings of this retrospective pilot study is questionable due to recall and participant biases, small sample size and the fact that there was no independent matched comparison group.

In an attempt to add to the available evidence regarding the effects of non-suturing, especially in relation to the long-term outcomes, Clement and Reed (1999) carried out a retrospective cohort study of women who had given birth in south-east London with unsutured perineal tears. Questionnaires were sent to women (n = 288) who had given birth between six months and seven years previously and had received care from a group of midwives (n = 5) who had been practising non-suturing for several years. Eighty percent of women responded (240/288) but only 107 who had tears which were unsutured were included in the analysis. Clement and Reed (1999) reported that very 'few women' were experiencing perineal pain at the time of completing the questionnaire and that generally they were 'very satisfied with having an unsutured perineal tear'. The researchers also reported that women (n = 20) who had experience of both sutured and non-sutured tears recalled that the sutured tear was more painful. The main conclusion drawn by Clement and Reed (1999) was that the findings of the study 'provide some evidence for the safety and acceptability of leaving some perineal tears unsutured'. However, it was difficult to interpret the results as there was no independent comparative group and there may have been participant recall bias. In addition, as acknowledged by the researchers themselves, 'women may have felt reticent about expressing dissatisfaction with the midwife who cared for them'.

The third study was a small retrospective audit carried out at the Crowborough birthing centre in the UK to assess the effects of not suturing second-degree tears (Wood, 1999). At eight weeks postpartum, the researcher asked fifty women (thirty-two primiparous and eighteen multiparous) 'if they were happy with the way their perineum had healed' and found that only one primiparous woman was not 'happy', reasons for which were not given.

The small randomised controlled trial which was carried out in Sweden by Lundquist *et al* (2000) compared non-suturing (n = 40) to suturing (n = 38) of spontaneous tears involving labia, vagina and perineum (included perineal tears which were not to exceed 2 x 2 cms). The trial recruited eighty primiparous women over an eighteen-month period from January 1996 to June 1997. Two women were excluded from the analysis because the midwife used non-absorbable instead of absorbable synthetic suture material. Outcomes were assessed at two to three days, eight weeks and six months postpartum. The researchers reported that more women (9/40 [23%]) in the non-suturing group described their perineal discomfort as a 'burning sensation' at two to three days postpartum compared with those (4/38 [11%]) in the sutured group. However, no differences were found in the rate of healing between the intervention groups up to six months following delivery. Data from this study must be interpreted with caution, as it is unclear how healing was defined and measured, the sample size was small and most of the results did not reach statistical significance.

More recently an RCT was carried out in Scotland to evaluate the short and long-term outcomes of non-suturing (n = 41) versus suturing (n = 33) (Fleming *et al*, 2003). Primiparous women with perineal lacerations following spontaneous birth were recruited into the trial from January 1999 to September 2000. Perineal pain and healing were assessed using standardised measures at one day, ten days and six weeks following birth. The trial found no significant difference in McGill pain scores at ten days or six weeks between groups, but reported that there was a statistically significant higher proportion of women at six weeks that had a closed tear in the sutured group (26/31 [84%]) compared to the non-sutured group (16/36 [44%]). As acknowledged by the trialists, it was impossible to blind the midwives assessing the trauma to the allocated treatment and this may have biased the results.

## Non-suturing of perineal skin

There is robust evidence from two large randomised controlled trials (RCTs) that show that there are no major adverse effects associated with leaving perineal skin unsutured (Gordon *et al*, 1998; Oboro *et al*, 2003). The trials carried out in the UK and Nigeria compared leaving the perineal skin unsutured but apposed (the vagina and perineal muscle were sutured) to the traditional repair whereby all three-layers (vagina, perineal muscles and skin) were sutured. Results relating to perineal pain were conflicting between trials. One of the RCTs carried out in a single centre in Ipswich, England (n = 1780 primiparous and multiparous women with first or second degree tears or episiotomies after spontaneous or assisted vaginal delivery) found no difference in short or long-term pain between the two groups (Gordon *et al*, 1998). However, the other RCT carried out in Nigeria (n = 823 women who sustained a second degree tear or episiotomy) found that leaving the skin unsutured was associated with a reduction in perineal pain up to three months postpartum (Oboro *et al*, 2003). The trials also reported lower rates of dyspareunia at three months postpartum in the groups that had the perineal skin left unsutured. Both trials found that leaving the perineal skin unsutured, but apposed, compared with suturing was associated with a significant increase in wound gaping at two days. The UK study found that the significant increase in wound gaping persisted in the non-sutured skin group up to ten days but the Nigerian study found a non-significant increase at fourteen days postpartum (Gordon *et al*, 1998; Oboro *et al*, 2003).

## Suture materials for primary perineal repair

Sutures have been used to close wounds throughout the ages with 'eyed' needles being invented somewhere between 50,000 and 30,000 BC (Mackenzie, 1973). The primary function of a suture is to maintain closure of the damaged tissue in order to promote healing by first intention, control bleeding and minimise the risk of infection. Wound edges must be approximated without tension otherwise the tissue will become devascularized and the healing process will be disrupted (Cuschieri *et al*, 2000).

The ideal suture material should cause minimal tissue reaction and be absorbed once it has served its purpose of holding the tissue in apposition during the healing process (Taylor and Karran, 1996). Well-aligned perineal wounds heal by primary intention with minimal complications, usually within two weeks of suturing. However, if the stitches remain in the tissues for longer than this period they act as a foreign body and may trigger a significant inflammatory response and impair healing. Once bacteria have colonised along the implanted sutures it is difficult to eradicate the infection and this may predispose to abscess formation and wound dehiscence. Local infection of the wound site will prolong the inflammatory phase and cause further tissue damage, which will delay collagen synthesis and epithelialization (Flanagan, 1997). Tissues with good blood supply, that heal rapidly and which are not under mechanical stress can be sutured with absorbable synthetic material. The two most common absorbable synthetic suture materials, which are used for perineal repair, are polyglycolic acid (Dexon, Davis & Geck Ltd, UK) and polyglactin 910 (Vicryl, Ethicon Ltd, Edinburgh, UK) which were introduced in 1970 and 1974 respectively.

A meta-analysis of eight randomised controlled trials (n = 3642 primiparous and multiparous women) that compared absorbable synthetic sutures (Dexon and Vicryl) to catgut suture material[1] found lower rates of perineal pain, analgesia use, suture dehiscence and resuturing in the Dexon and Vicryl groups (Kettle and Johanson, 2004). However, there was no clear difference in terms of long-term pain and dyspareunia between the intervention groups. Two of the trials (n = 2129 women) found that Dexon and Vicryl were associated with an increased risk of suture removal up to three months postpartum (Mahomed *et al*, 1989; Mackrodt *et al*, 1998).

More recently, a new type of polyglactin 910 suture material (Vicryl Rapide) has become available for perineal repair which has the same chemical composition as standard Vicryl but it is absorbed in less time due to a change in the sterilisation process using gamma irradiation. The tensile strength (breaking strength) of Vicryl Rapide is reduced at ten to fourteen days and it is completely absorbed from the tissue by forty-two days (Ethicon, 1991). There have been one prospective cohort study and three randomised controlled trials undertaken to evaluate rapidly absorbed polyglactin 910 suture material (Vicryl Rapide) for perineal repair to date (Masson *et al*, 1988; Gemynthe *et*

---

1   Catgut suture material has been withdrawn from the UK market since 2002.

*al*, 1996; McElhinney *et al*, 2000, Kettle *et al*, 2002).

The cohort study (n = 2000 women who sustained an episiotomy or tear) undertaken in France by Masson *et al* (1988) investigated the effects of rapidly absorbed polyglactin 910 suture material (Vicryl Rapide). Vaginal trauma was repaired using a 'continuous technique' and interrupted sutures were inserted to close the perineal muscles and skin. Results from the study showed a 2% rate (n = 40) of wound dehiscence at day three postpartum, which was attributed to the 'saw-through' effect of interrupted transcutaneous stitches tied too tightly. They also reported that 99% (n = 1979) of the participants had 'no pain' at day six postpartum and that the patients could not 'pinpoint' the date of suture disappearance. Only three women had wounds with poor cosmetic results, one of which required secondary intervention.

Gemynthe *et al* (1996) carried out a randomised controlled trial (n = 308 primiparous women) in Denmark to assess the effects of rapidly absorbed polyglactin 910 suture material (Vicryl Rapide). The main outcome measures were perineal pain and wound dehiscence. Women with an episiotomy (n = 145) or tear (n = 163) were randomly allocated to receive rapidly absorbed polyglactin 910 (n = 155) or standard polyglactin 910 material (n = 153). The trauma was sutured as routine with subcuticular sutures inserted to appose the superficial layer of the perineum. Results from the trial showed no difference in the overall amount of short and long-term pain between materials but there was a significant reduction in pain at day fourteen 'when walking' in the rapidly absorbed polyglactin 910 group, 33.3% (n = 46) as compared with 48.5% (n = 65) in the standard polyglactin 910 group. Approximately 60% of women in each group reported recommencing sexual intercourse before twelve weeks postpartum and approximately two-thirds of these complained of dyspareunia. There was no significant difference in suture removal between groups at eight weeks postpartum and insufficient healing was reported by 6% (n = 9) of women in both groups. The researchers concluded that a larger study was needed to explore these results further.

McElhinney and colleagues fron Northern Ireland (2000) carried out the second randomised controlled trial, to compare the effects of rapidly absorbed polyglactin 910 suture material (Vicryl Rapide) (n = 75) to standard material (Vicryl) (n = 78). The main outcome measures were perineal pain, dyspareunia, wound problems and suture removal. Women (primiparous and multiparous) who sustained a tear or episiotomy following spontaneous vaginal delivery were randomly allocated to the intervention or control groups. Operators repaired the trauma with one length of suture material using the 'same technique' and subcuticular stitches to close the perineal skin. All participating women received a diclofenac suppository (100mgs) per rectum following perineal repair for pain relief. Women were recruited into the trial over a six-month period from February to July 1996, and 77% of the participants completed follow-up at six and twelve weeks postpartum. The participants were interviewed twenty-four hours following delivery and a clinical examination and interview were carried out on day three. At six and twelve weeks women were contacted via telephone regarding outcomes relating to sexual dysfunction. In addition, the general practitioner/family doctor or obstetrician assessed the participants during their postnatal check-up with regard to healing complications. The trial found that there was no difference in pain up to three days postpartum between suture materials but, at six weeks, a significant reduction in dyspareunia was reported by women in the rapidly absorbed polyglactin 910 group (Vicryl Rapide) (denominators not presented in paper). They also reported that 30% of women sutured with standard polyglactin 910 (Vicryl) material experienced wound problems such as dehiscence, pain or removal of suture material as compared with 1.7% in the rapidly absorbed polyglactin 910 group (Vicryl Rapide). At twelve weeks postpartum, 20% of women in the standard polyglactin 910 group (Vicryl) reported dyspareunia as compared to 5% in the rapidly absorbed polyglactin 910 group (Vicryl Rapide). However, these findings must be interpreted with caution due to the small number of participants in each group. A larger study or meta-analysis of smaller studies is needed to explore these results further.

The third large factorial randomised controlled trial was carried out in the UK by Kettle *et al* (2002) to evaluate the short and long-term effects of rapidly absorbed polyglactin 910 suture material (Vicryl Rapide) (n = 772) to standard polyglactin 910 suture material (Vicryl) (n = 770) and to either the continuous (n = 771) or interrupted (n = 771) suturing method. The main outcome measures were perineal pain, superficial dyspareunia and suture removal. All women (primiparous and multiparous) who had a spontaneous vaginal delivery were randomly allocated to receive one of the treatments and the perineal repair was carried out by one of the participating midwives (n = 150). Recruitment into the trial took place over a nineteen-month period from June 1997 to December 1998 and 90% of the participants completed follow-up at twelve months postpartum. Both women and midwives completed questionnaires independently at two and ten days postpartum and women were also sent a postal questionnaire at three and twelve months after birth. Results from the trial showed no significant difference in short or long-term pain, wound dehiscence or dyspareunia. However, there was a statistically significant reduction in pain when 'walking' in the Vicryl Rapide group (n = 259/769 [33.7%]) compared to the standard Vicryl group (n = 314/770 [40.8%]), which mirrors the findings of the small study by Gemynthe *et al* (1996). The trial also found that suture removal was significantly less in the Vicryl Rapide group (n = 22/769 [2.7%]) compared to the standard Vicryl group (n = 98/770 [12.7%]) up to three months postpartum.

In summary, all three randomised controlled trials (n = 2003 women) found no clear difference in short-term pain between Vicryl Rapide and standard Vicryl (Gemynthe *et al*, 1996; McElhinney *et al*, 2000; Kettle *et al*, 2002). Two of the trials (n = 1850 women) found a significant reduction in 'pain when walking' at ten to fourteen days postpartum (Gemynthe *et al*, 1996; Kettle *et al*, 2002). Only one of the trials (n = 153 women) reported a reduction in superficial dyspareunia at three months postpartum (McElhinney *et al*, 2000). All three randomised controlled trials found that Vicryl Rapide suture material was associated with a significant reduction in the need for suture removal up to three months following childbirth (Gemynthe *et al*, 1996; McElhinney *et al*, 2000; Kettle *et al*, 2002). Previous research has found that absorbable synthetic suture materials (Dexon and Vicryl) compared to catgut is associated with a reduction in perineal pain, but one of the main concerns was the need to remove Dexon and Vicryl sutures up to three months following delivery (Kettle and Johanson, 2004). For every ten women whose repair was undertaken with Vicryl Rapide suture material, one less had discomfort from suture removal. Therefore, current evidence supports Vicryl Rapide as the most appropriate suture material for primary perineal repair.

## Suture methods for primary perineal repair

Perineal trauma is usually repaired in three stages. First, a continuous locking stitch is inserted to close vaginal trauma, commencing at the apex of the wound and finishing at the level of the fourchette with a loop knot. The rationale for using a locking stitch is to prevent shortening of the vagina but there is no good quality evidence to support this. Next, the deep and superficial muscles are re-approximated with three or four interrupted sutures or sometimes a continuous 'running' stitch. Finally, the skin is closed using a continuous subcutaneous technique or interrupted transcutaneous sutures are inserted. However, many midwives and students are taught to suture using the interrupted method because it is considered easier to learn and may cause fewer problems in the hands of the inexperienced or novice operator (Grant, 1989).

## Perineal skin closure

Meta-analysis of four randomised controlled trials (n = 1681 primiparous and multiparous women) found that a continuous subcuticular technique for perineal skin closure, when compared to interrupted transcutaneous stitches, was associated with less short-term pain (Kettle and Johanson, 2004). Three of the trials (n = 1588) presented data on pain up to ten days in a suitable format for inclusion in the analysis (Banninger *et al*, 1978; Isager-Sally *et al*, 1986; Mahomed *et al*, 1989) and only one study (Isager-Sally *et al*, 1986) actually demonstrated any statistical significance between the two treatment groups. Two of the included trials (n = 1068) presented data relating to analgesia use in the immediate postpartum period but no differences were seen between groups (Banninger *et al*, 1978 and Mahomed *et al*, 1989). One trial (n = 916 women) presented data regarding long-term pain, which found a non-significant increase in the continuous subcuticular group (Mahomed *et al*, 1989). Only three of the trials (n = 1524) provided data regarding the extent of reported dyspareunia up to three months following birth which showed that there was no statistically significant difference between the groups (Detlefsen *et al*, 1980; Isager-Sally *et al*, 1986; Mahomed *et al*, 1989). One trial (n = 916) reported that sutures were removed less frequently up to three months postpartum in the continuous subcuticular group compared to the interrupted group (Mahomed *et al*, 1989).

## Continuous non-locking technique

For more than seventy years researchers have been suggesting that continuous suture techniques of perineal repair are far better than interrupted methods in terms of reduced postpartum pain and yet they have not been generally used (Rucker, 1930; Mandy *et al*, 1951; Christhilf and Monias, 1962; Guilhem *et al*, 1960; Detlefsen *et al*, 1980; Isager-Sally *et al*, 1986; Fleming, 1990; Olah, 1994).

In 1930 Rucker first reported using a continuous running stitch for repair of episiotomies or tears using silk-worm gut suture material to appose the deep tissues and superficial subcutaneous layer (Rucker, 1930). A continuous longitudinal mattress stitch was inserted to appose the vagina and 'levator fibres' and then a second row of sutures were inserted parallel to the first layer. Using this technique, the perineum was built up layer by layer with approximately four rows of sutures being inserted. Rucker reported that the patients were more comfortable following repair with this technique and the 'results were uniformly excellent'. The repair was completed by a continuous stitch to close the superficial submucous and subcutaneous tissues.

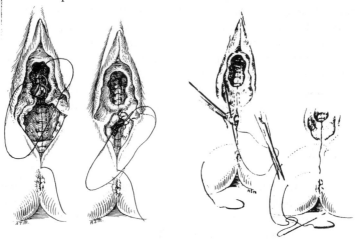

**Figure 4.2: Rucker technique of perineal repair**

## Underlying theory

With the continuous suture technique there are no knots and 'the sutures accommodate themselves to the swelling as it occurs'. There is also no 'cutting' of the tissues by the stitches. Rucker thought that it was difficult to know just exactly how tight or loose to tie interrupted sutures in order to allow for reactionary tissue swelling. He postulated that if the sutures were tied too loosely then 'primary union' would not be achieved and if they were tied too tightly they were inclined to cut into the tissues and cause increased pain when swelling occurred. He also stated that when transverse interrupted sutures were used, often only the outer part of the wound was repaired which resulted in a 'shallow perinei or so-called "dash-board" perineum'. In contrast, when longitudinal continuous sutures were used to repair the trauma in layers the perineum felt 'thick and firm'.

In order to determine if the 'Rucker' technique would reduce postpartum pain, when compared with other methods, Mandy *et al* (1951) studied 200 'cases of perineal repairs'. One hundred cases were repaired using the 'Rucker' technique and a further 100 were repaired as routine with No.00 chromic catgut suture material by obstetricians and general practitioners at the Franklin Square Hospital, Baltimore. The researchers reported on day four that 83/100 (83%) of women who were repaired using the 'Rucker' technique experienced no discomfort and required no pain relief medication as compared to 23/100 (23%) who had other methods. Indeed, most women who had the 'Rucker' repair were unaware of having stitches and typically responded when questioned about perineal pain, 'Do I have stitches?' The operators found that this method was not technically difficult to perform; it could be used on median as well as medio-lateral episiotomies and that the additional few minutes spent on the repair

In 1990 Fleming published her experience of using a simple non-locking, continuous suturing technique for all layers, with subcutaneous stitches placed well below the perineal skin surface. Previous research has highlighted the technical difficulty of carrying out subcuticular suturing but Fleming reported that the continuous method was easy to perform and could be easily taught to relatively inexperienced operators (Fleming 1993, personal communication). She was taught this method by an obstetrician named William Schafer (her husband) with whom she worked in private by Christhilf and Monias on a series of 350 cases over a twenty-four-month period (Christhilf and Monias, 1962). The modification involved abandoning the four-layer closure for a three-layer repair using a finer catgut material and a 'swedged-on needle'. A single suture length of chromic catgut 2/0, which had a half circle taper needle on one end and a straight cutting needle on the other was used to facilitate the repair.

The suturing was commenced at the lower end of the perineal wound instead of the apex of the vaginal mucosa and a continuous running stitch was used to re-approximate the deep and superficial tissues instead of the longitudinal mattress stitch, which was used in the original 'Rucker' method. In addition, a continuous transcutaneous locked suture was used to appose the vaginal trauma instead of a submucosal stitch. Once the repair was complete, the two ends of the suture material were brought out separately through the skin, well away from the wound edges and then cut off level with the skin surface.

Assessment of this technique by Christhilf and Monias (1962) was based purely on clinical impression and they made no attempt to repeat statistical evaluation of the procedure. Perineal assessment was made at the time of discharge from the hospital on the fourth or fifth day following delivery and the results were reported to be 'mutually satisfactory to the patient and obstetrician'. Many of the patients were surprised that they had stitches and 'contrasted the results favourably against previous experiences'. Christhilf and Monias (1962) found that the continuous technique was rapid to perform, there were no significant infections, postpartum discomfort was minimal, healing was always by first intention and there were no wound breakdown or fistulae. Indeed, one wonders why the Rucker method never achieved more widespread knowledge or acceptance and why it was not described in textbooks.

In 1990, Fleming published her experience of using a simple non-locking, continuous suturing technique for all layers, with subcutaneous stitches placed well below the perineal skin surface. Previous research has highlighted the technical difficulty of carrying out subcuticular suturing but Fleming reported that the continuous method was easy to perform and could be easily taught to relatively inexperienced operators (Fleming, 1993, personal communication). She was taught this method by an obstetrician named William Schafer (her husband) with whom she worked in private practice.

The basic premise of this 'alternative' technique is that the sutures are placed 'loose and deep' in as few layers as possible to reduce the amount of foreign material implanted in the wound. The repair begins with an anchoring stitch above the apex of the vaginal trauma and the deep tissues and mucosa are closed with a single continuous 'running' stitch in comparison to the 'locking' stitch, which Christhilf and Monias used. Next, the deep and superficial perineal muscles are re-approximated with a continuous, loose non-locking stitch, with care taken to occlude the 'dead space'. The repair is completed with a continuous suture inserted well below the skin surface in the subcutaneous fascia to avoid the 'profusion of nerve endings' and is finished off with a terminal knot placed in the vagina. A single length of absorbable suture material is used for the repair with no knots other than the anchoring and terminal knot. Fleming reported that the 'alternative repair technique results in a skin-edge gap of 2 to 3 mm' which initially caused some 'personal uneasiness' regarding a possible increased risk of wound infection and the 'long-term cosmetic results'.

Fleming (1987) found surprisingly low levels of pain reported by women who were sutured with the loose continuous method 'compared to general expectations and reports from other researchers' when more traditional suture methods were used. By forty-eight hours postpartum the mean perceived perineal pain in both the laceration and episiotomy groups was rated as mild and by two weeks the women reported having virtually no pain (Fleming, 1987). At six weeks postpartum good cosmetic results were found on clinical examination and the scar was reported to be only of hairline thickness (Fleming, 1990).

The underlying principles of this 'alternative' loose continuous technique as described by Fleming in a later paper (1990) appear to be based on the method used by Christhilf and Monias (1962). However, Fleming was unaware of any of the previous work that had been carried out to evaluate continuous suturing techniques of perineal repair (Fleming 2002, personal communication). In summary, the 'alternative' continuous suturing technique appears to be associated with a lower incidence of pain compared with the results from other research studies using more traditional methods of perineal repair (Fleming, 1990). However, Fleming's findings were based purely on an observational study and not a randomised controlled comparative trial.

More recently, the large factorial randomised controlled trial (n = 1542 women) designed by Kettle and colleagues (2002) to build on previous research, compared the loose non-locking continuous technique as described by Fleming (1990) to the more traditional interrupted method of perineal repair (details of the trial have been described previously on *page 43*). Results showed a significant reduction in perineal pain at ten days when the loose continuous technique was used for all layers (204/770 [26.5%]) compared with the interrupted method (338/769 [44.0%]). For every six women who were sutured with the continuous technique there was one less who complained of pain at ten days compared to those sutured with the interrupted method. The reduction in reported pain in the continuous suture group (31/700 [4.4%]) compared to the interrupted group (47/689 [6.4%]) persisted up to twelve months after childbirth but did not reach statistical significance. Women reported no difference in superficial dyspareunia at three months (amongst those who had resumed intercourse) between the intervention groups (98/581 [16.9%]) in the continuous group compared with 102/593 [17.2%] in the interrupted group). Suture removal was significantly less frequent in the continuous suturing group (24/770 [3.0%]) compared with the interrupted group (96/769 [12.0%]) up to three months following birth.

It is interesting to note that women who were allocated to the non-locking continuous suturing technique of perineal repair stated that 'they did not know that they had sutures' which was a similar response to that made by women who had the 'Rucker' method of repair. Furthermore, as reported by Fleming (1990) the midwives performing the continuous suturing technique found that it was not technically difficult to perform. Another benefit of continuous suturing is that only one piece of suture material is required to complete the perineal repair as compared to two or three for the interrupted method, thus reducing overall expenditure.

It can, therefore, be concluded from the current research evidence that perineal trauma should be repaired using the continuous non-locking technique to re-approximate all layers (vagina, perineal muscles and skin) with Vicryl Rapide suture material. All health professionals responsible for carrying out perineal repairs should receive appropriate training to ensure that they are able to recognise the extent of trauma sustained and to enable skilful repair of perineal injuries following birth. Women who explicitly request not to have perineal trauma sutured must be given the opportunity to discuss their concerns with the person providing care. The person responsible for the woman's care should thoroughly inspect the perineal trauma, using good lighting and the full extent of injury should be carefully documented in the hospital case notes. If the woman does not wish to be examined it is essential to discuss potential risks with her, such as anal incontinence, which may occur if trauma to the sphincters remains undetected.

## Main principles of perineal repair

Regardless of suturing method used the following basic surgical principles should be applied:

- ⌘ Carry out the perineal suturing as soon as possible following the birth to minimise the risk of infection and blood loss.
- ⌘ Prior to commencing the suturing check all equipment and count the number of swabs. This should be repeated once the operator has finished the procedure.
- ⌘ Perineal tears and episiotomies should be repaired under aseptic conditions.
- ⌘ A good source of light is necessary to enable the operator to visualise the full extent of injury and to identify the structures involved.
- ⌘ Ensure that appropriate supervision or support is available prior to commencing the repair and, if in doubt regarding the extent of trauma or structures involved, ask for more experienced assistance.
- ⌘ Complex trauma should be repaired in theatre under regional or general anaesthesia by an experienced operator. An indwelling catheter should be inserted for twenty-four hours to prevent urinary retention.
- ⌘ Perineal tissue should be handled gently using non-toothed forceps.
- ⌘ The dead space should be closed to ensure good haemostasis to prevent haematoma formation and infection.
- ⌘ The minimal amount of suture material should be inserted.
- ⌘ It is important not to over-tighten sutures as this may cause tissue hypoxia and delay healing.
- ⌘ Sutures should be tied securely but not too bulky using a square surgeon's knot.
- ⌘ It is important to ensure that good anatomical restoration of the perineal tissues is achieved and consideration given to the finished cosmetic results.
- ⌘ Following completion of the repair an accurate detailed account of the repair should be documented plus the method and materials used (black ink, print and sign name). It is useful to include a diagram to illustrate the extent of the trauma.

✻ The person responsible for the perineal repair should inform the woman regarding:
  - extent of trauma
  - methods of pain relief
  - dietary considerations
  - the importance of rest
  - personal hygiene
  - pelvic floor exercises
  - avoidance of constipation.
✻ The woman should be given information regarding who to contact if problems such as superficial dyspareunia or urinary or faecal incontinence persists. It is important that women are encouraged to report any problems sooner rather than later to enable prompt sensitive care to be initiated that is both appropriate and effective.

## Basic surgical skills

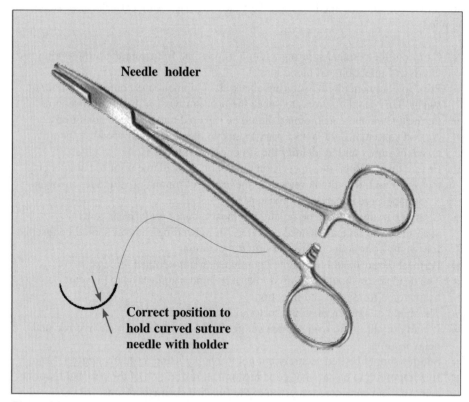

**Figure 4.3: Correct positioning of needle onto holder**

## Using dissecting forceps

Dissecting forceps should be held in the non-dominant hand and used instead of fingers to facilitate positioning of the suturing needle onto the needle holder (*Figure 4.4a*); to steady the needle when it emerges from the tissue (*Figure 4.4b*), and to manipulate tissue during the repair (*Figure 4.5c*).

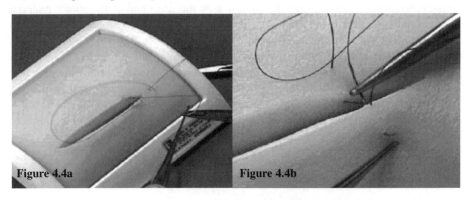

Figure 4.4a  Figure 4.4b

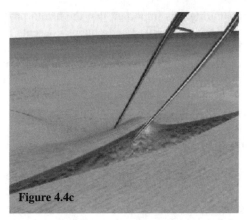

Figure 4.4c

## Tying surgeons square knots with instruments

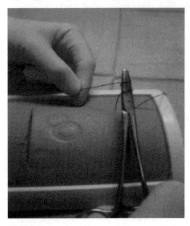

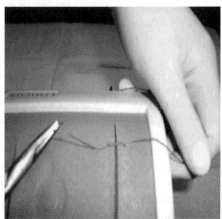

Insert the first suture by taking a bite on the first side of the wound ensuring that the needle follows the line of its curvature. The needle is removed and re-positioned in the needle holder using the dissecting forceps (held in the non-dominant hand) before taking another bite on the opposite side of the wound. Pull the suture through so that the free end is fairly short. Next, the end of the suture material with needle attached is looped twice around the needle holder (this prevents the second throw slipping and over-tightening) and the instrument's jaws grasps the short end of the suture material and it is pulled tight, ensuring that the first throw lies flat. The second throw reverses the direction of the suture material around the needle holder and also the direction by which the hands pull the suture material when tightening the throw to ensure that a square surgeon's knot (reef knot) is made. A third throw is made changing the direction of the suture material around the needle holder and also the direction by which the hands pull the suture material. The suture material is then pulled outwards and upwards to secure the knot. Either the shirt end is cut if the stitch is an anchoring suture or both ends are cut if it is a single interrupted stitch.

## Procedure for perineal repair

Prior to commencing suturing it is important that the health professional explains the procedure to the woman and her partner and obtains consent. The woman should be placed in a comfortable position so that the trauma is easily visualised. Good lighting is essential. It is vital to perform a rectal examination as routine when assessing perineal injury after delivery to avoid missing trauma to the anal sphincters (internal or external). This should be repeated once the repair is complete to ensure that suture material has not been accidentally inserted through the rectal mucosa.

### Identification of anal sphincter injury:

- Look for absence of anal 'puckering' around the anterior aspect of the anus (between 9 and 3 o'clock).
- Observe if the perineal trauma extends down to the anal margin.
- Insert your index finger into the woman's anus and ask her to squeeze (explain to the woman why this is necessary and obtain her consent prior to performing the examination). If the external anal sphincter is torn, the separated ends can be observed to retract backwards towards the ischiorectal fossa.
- Damage to the internal anal sphincter is more difficult to detect.

It is not necessary to use lithotomy poles to support the woman's legs during the procedure. Restraining the woman's legs may bring back locked in memories of sexual abuse in some women and could make others feel helpless, out of control and undignified. There is no need to use a tampon. If the woman is breast-feeding 'skin to skin' contact can be maintained throughout the procedure if it is the mother's wish.

Follow the basic surgical principles throughout the procedure as documented above and clean the perineal area according to local policy. Ensure that the wound is adequately anaesthetised (10–20mls Lignocaine 1%). Inject local anaesthetic into the traumatised tissue ensuring even distribution. Check that the perineal area is adequately anaesthetised prior to commencing the repair and, if necessary, administer more local anaesthetic. It is important to note that women may forget the pain of childbirth but will never forget the pain associated with 'stitches'.

## The continuous suturing technique

The continuous suturing technique is illustrated below. The first stitch is inserted above the apex of the vaginal trauma to secure any bleeding points that might not be visible. Vaginal trauma, perineal muscle (deep and superficial) and skin are re-approximated with a loose, non-locking continuous technique.

### Step 1— suturing the vagina

❖ Identify the apex.
❖ Check if the trauma is bilateral or unilateral.
❖ Insert first stitch above apex to secure any bleeding points.
❖ Close the vaginal trauma with a loose continuous stitch.
❖ Make sure each bite is not too wide as this may cause narrowing of the vagina.
❖ Continue to suture down to hymenal remnants.
❖ Insert the needle through the skin at the fourchette to emerge in the centre of the perineal trauma.

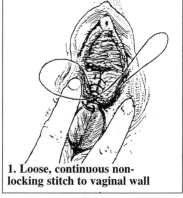

**1. Loose, continuous non-locking stitch to vaginal wall**

### Step 2 — suturing the muscle layer

❖ Check the depth of the trauma.
❖ Close the perineal muscle using a continuous non-locking stitch.
❖ If necessary, insert two layers of sutures.
❖ Take care not to leave any dead space.
❖ Ensure that stitches are not inserted through into the rectum or anal canal.
❖ Re-align muscle so that the skin edges can be brought together without any tension.

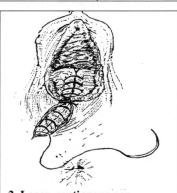

**2. Loose, continuous non-locking stitch to perineal muscles**

### Step 3 — *suturing the perineal skin*

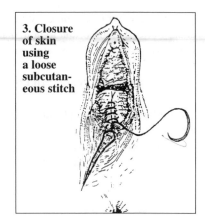

**3. Closure of skin using a loose subcutaneous stitch**

❖ At the inferior end of the wound bring needle out under the skin surface, reversing the stitching direction.
❖ Stitches are placed below the skin surface in the subcutaneous layer thus avoiding the profusion of nerve endings.
❖ Continue taking bites of tissue from each side of the wound until the hymenal remnants are reached.
❖ Secure the finished repair with a loop or Aberdeen knot in the vagina.

## Finally

❖ Check that the finished repair is anatomically correct and there is no excessive bleeding.
❖ Perform a vaginal examination and check that two fingers can easily be inserted and that the vagina has not been stitched too tight.
❖ Carry out a rectal examination to ensure no sutures have been inserted into the rectal mucosa. If sutures are inserted by mistake a recto-vaginal fistulae may occur if the stitches are not removed.
❖ Check that all swabs, needles and instruments are correct.
❖ Place the woman in a comfortable position.
❖ Complete documentation to fulfil the statutory requirements and to provide an accurate account of the repair.

## Repair of third and fourth degree tears

Third and fourth degree tears must be repaired by an experienced practitioner who has received specialised training and is competent to carry out the procedure. All repairs should be carried out under general or spinal anaesthetic in an operating theatre with good lighting, and appropriate equipment. Currently, there are no randomised controlled trials to provide reliable evidence regarding the best method or material for repair of the third and fourth degree tears.

### Torn anal epithelium or rectal mucosa

Torn anal epithelium or rectal mucosa is repaired with 3/0 gauge absorbable synthetic material using either interrupted stitches (the knots should be tied in the anal lumen) or a continuous submucosal stitch.

## Torn internal anal sphincter

If the internal anal sphincter is torn this must be repaired separately by end-to-end approximation with 3/0 gauge monofilament suture material such as Polydioxanone (Ethicon Ltd) using interrupted stitches.

## Torn external anal sphincter

If the external anal sphincter is torn more than 50% it is repaired using either the overlap or end-to-end technique according to the operator's preference. If a 3a (less than 50%) tear is sustained the torn fibres are repaired using the end-to-end technique. The torn ends are repaired with 3/0 gauge monofilament suture material such as Polydioxanone (Ethicon Ltd).

### *Overlap technique*

The torn ends of the external anal sphincter are overlapped (double breast fashion) and sutured with interrupted stitches.

### *End-to-end technique*

Th torn ends of the external anal sphincter are re-approximated end-to-end and sutured with interrupted sutures (conventional mattress sutures).

## Torn vaginal, perineal muscles and perineal skin

Following the repair of the anal epithelium, rectal mucosa, internal and external anal sphincter (depending on the degree of trauma sustained), the vagina, perineal muscles and skin are repaired as described above using absorbable synthetic material (Vicryl Rapide).

Following completion of the repair it is important to record accurately in the medical notes, details of the anatomical structures involved, classification of the injury, method of repair, suture materials used and all swabs, instruments and sharps were accounted for. It is useful to include a diagram to illustrate the extent of damage sustained.

## Management

Mismanagement of third and fourth degree perineal trauma is associated with a significant amount of postpartum morbidity. Midwives and medical staff must be aware of this type of severe trauma and be adequately trained to identify anal sphincter injuries when they occur. Short-term problems include perineal pain, increased risk of infection and wound dehiscence, while long-term complications include anal incontinence (defined as loss of flatus, liquid and solid faeces). Obstetric anal sphincter damage, if missed at the time of delivery or managed inappropriately, is a potential source of litigation.

It is important that the woman is given a full explanation of the injury sustained and a contact number to ring if she has any problems during the postnatal period. Follow-up should be available at specialist clinics for up to twelve months postpartum or longer if necessary so that problems can be promptly identified and effectively treated. Best practice suggests that women with persistent anal problems should be referred for anal manometry, ultrasound scan, and consultation with a colorectal surgeon.

## The international perspective

It is imperative that women receive high quality evidence-based care relating to the management and repair of perineal trauma wherever childbirth takes place. Furthermore, practitioners should receive appropriate structured training in the identification, classification and repair of perineal trauma in order to minimise both the short and long-term maternal morbidity associated with this procedure if carried out perfunctorily. Most research relating to methods and materials used for perineal repair has been undertaken in developed countries; however, the results are generalisable and should be implemented by practitioners worldwide. For example, the simple and widely practicable continuous perineal repair technique prevented one woman in six from experiencing pain at ten days postpartum. Moreover, for every ten women who were repaired with more rapidly absorbed polyglactin 910 (Vicryl Rapide) suture material, one less was spared the pain and unpleasantness of having perineal sutures removed. Implementation of evidence-based practices that reduce the adverse sequelae of perineal trauma and make vaginal birth more desirable should be encouraged. This will not only improve maternal morbidity for women throughout the world but may also decrease the escalating interest in caesarean section as an alternative mode of delivery.

## References

Aljafri AM, Kingsnorth A (1998) *Fundamentals of Surgical Practice*. 1st edn. Greenwich Medical Media Limited, London

Ashcroft GS, Dodsworth J, van Boxtel E, Tarnuzzer RW, Horan MA, Schultz GS, Ferguson MW (1997) Estrogen accelerates cutaneous wound healing associated with an increase in TGF-beta levels. *Nature Med* 3(11): 1209–15

Banninger U, Buhrig H, Schreiner WE (1978) [A comparison between chromic catgut and polyglycolic acid sutures in episiotomy repair]. *Geburtshilfe Frauenheilkd* 33: 30–33

Brimacombe J (1995) Reaping the pain which others have sewn. *The Independent*, 14 March: 21

Cain JJ, Shirar E (1996) A new method for teaching the repair of perineal trauma at birth. *Fam Med* 28(2): 107–10

Clement S, Reed B (1999) To stitch or not to stitch? A long term follow up study of women with unsutured perineal tears. *Practising Midwife* 2(4): 20–8

Carroli G, Belizan JM (2002) *Episiotomy for vaginal birth*. Cochrane Review. In: The Cochrane Library, Issue 1. Update Software, Oxford

Christhilf SM, Monias MB (1962) Knotless episiorrhaphy as a positive approach towards eliminating postpartum perineal distress. *Am J Obstet Gynecol* 84(6): 812–8

Coats PM, Chan KK, Wilkins M, Beard RJ (1980) A comparison between midline and mediolateral episiotomies. *Br J Obstet Gynaecol* **87**: 409–12

Cuschieri A, Steele RJC, Moossa AR (2000) *Essential Surgical Practice*. 4th edn. Butterworth-Heinemann, Oxford

Derry DE (1935) Note on five pelves of women of the Eleventh Dynasty in Egypt. *J Obstet Gynaecol of the British Empire* **xiii**: 490–5

Detlefsen GU, Vinther S, Larsen P, Schroeder E (1980) [Intradermal suturing of episiotomy wounds compared with interrupted sutures]. *Ugeskr Laeger* **142**: 3117–20

Dyer C (2001) Bristol inquiry condemns hospital's 'club culture'. *Br Med J* **323**: 181

Eccles A (1982) *Obstetrics and Gynaecology in Tudor and Stuart England*. 1st edn. Croom Helm Ltd, London

Ethicon (1991) *A unique new product completes the family: VICRYL rapide*. Ethicon Limited, Edinburgh

Flanagan M (1997) *Wound Management*. Churchill Livingstone, Edinburgh

Fleming N (1987) *Comparison of Women with Different Perineal Conditions after Childbirth*. Ann Arbor, Michigan UMI

Fleming N (1990) Can the suturing method make a difference in postpartum perineal pain? *J Nurse-Midwifery* **35**(1): 19–25

Fleming EM, Hagen S, Niven C (2003) Does perineal suturing make a difference? The SUNS trial. *Br J Obstet Gynaecol* **110**: 684–9

Foster D (2002) *The Dr Foster Good Birth Guide*. Vermilion, London

Gemynthe A, Langhoff-Roos J, Sahl S, Knudsen J (1996) New VICRYL formulation: an improved method of perineal repair? *Br J Midwif* **4**(5): 230–4

Graham H (1950) *Eternal Eve*. William Heinemann Medical Books Ltd, Britain

Grant A (1989) Repair of perineal trauma after childbirth. In: Chalmers I, Enkin M, Keirse MJMC, eds. *Effective Care in Pregnancy and Childbirth*. Oxford University Press, Oxford: 1179–81

Greenshileds W, Hulme H (1993) *The Perineum in Childbirth: A survey of women's experiences and midwifery practices*. National Childbirth Trust, London

Gordon B, Mackrodt C, Fern E, Truesdale A, Ayers S, Grant A (1998) The Ipswich Childbirth Study: 1. A randomised evaluation of two-stage postpartum perineal repair leaving the skin unsutured. *Br J Obstet Gynaecol* **104**(4): 435–40

Guilhem P, Pontonnier A, Espagno G (1960) [Episiotomie prophylactique. Suture intradermique.] *Gynécologie et Obstétrique* 59(2): 261–7

Head M (1993) Dropping stitches. *Nurs Times* **89**(33): 64–5

Hogston P (2001) Suture choice in general gynaecological surgery. *The Obstetrician and Gynaecologist* **3**(3): 127–31

Isager-Sally L, Legarth J, Jacobsen B, Bostofte E (1986) Episiotomy repair — immediate and long-term sequelae. A prospective randomized study of three different methods of repair. *Br J Obstet Gynaecol* **93**: 420–5

Jelovsek FR (1995) A guest editorial. Teaching basic skills in obs-gyn. *Obstet Gynecol Surv* **50**(9): 633

Kettle C, Johanson RB (2004) *Absorbable synthetic versus catut suture material for perineal repair* (Cochrane Review). In: The Cochrane Library, Issue 3. Update Software, Oxford

Kettle C, Hills RK, Jones P *et al* (2002) Continuous versus interrupted perineal repair with standard or rapidly absorbed sutures after spontaneous vaginal birth: a randomised controlled trial. *Lancet* **359**: 2217–23

Klein MC, Gauthier RJ, Robbins JM, Kaczorowski J, Jorgensen SH, Franco ED *et al* (1994) Relationship of episiotomy to perineal trauma and morbidity, sexual dysfunction and pelvic floor relaxation. *Am J Obstet Gynecol* **71**: 591–8

Koopmann CF (1995) Cutaneous wound healing. *Otolaryngol Clin North Am* **28**(5): 835–45

Krueger JK, Rohrich RJ (2001) Clearing the smoke: the scientific rationale for tobacco abstention with plastic surgery. *Plast Reconst Surg* **108**(4): 1063–73

Larsson PG, Platz-Christensen JJ, Bergman B, Wallstersson G (1991) Advantage or disadvantage of episiotomy compared with spontaneous perineal laceration. *Gynecologic Obstetric Investigation* **31**(4): 213–6

Lewis L (1994) Are you sitting comfortably? The development of a perineal audit system to enable midwives to follow their perineal management up to thirteen months postnatally. *Midwives Chronicle*: 226–7

Lundquist M, Olsson A, Nissen E, Norman M (2000) Is it necessary to suture all lacerations after vaginal delivery? *Birth* **27**(2); 79–85

Mackenzie D (1973) The history of sutures. *History of Medicine* **17**: 158

Mackrodt C, Gordon B, Fern E, Ayers S, Truesdale A, Grant A (1998) The Ipswich Childbirth study: 2. A randomised comparison of polyglactin 910 with chromic catgut for postpartum perineal repair. *Br J Obstet Gynaecol* **105**(4): 441–5

Magdi I (1949) Obstetric injuries of the perineum. *Journal of Obstetrics and Gynaecology of the British Commonwealth* **49**: 687–700

Masson F, Bilweis J, Di Lucca D, Trentesaux G, Wrobe N (1988) Interest in a new suture material for 2000 episiotomy repairs: Polyglactin 910. *Clinique Gynécologique et Obstétricale*: 19–21

McElhinney BR, Glenn DRJ, harper MA (2000) Episiotomy repair: vicryl versus vicryl rapide. *The Ulster Medical Journal* **69**(1): 27–9

McGuiness M, Norr K, Nacion K (1991) Comparison between different perineal outcomes on tissue healing. *J Nurse-Midwifery* **36**(3): 192–8

Mandel LP, Lentz GM, Goff BA (2000) Teaching and evaluating surgical skills. *Obstet Gynecol* **95**(5): 783–5

Mikhailidis DP, Barradas MA, Jeremy JY, Dandona P (1983) Cigarette smoking inhibits prostacyclin formation. *Lancet* **2**(8350): 627–8

Mahomed K, Grant A, Ashurst H, James D (1989) The Southmead perineal suture study. A randomized comparison of suture materials and suturing materials and suturing techniques for repair of perineal trauma. *Br J Obstet Gynaecol* **96**: 1272–80

Mandy TE, Christhilf SM, Mandy AJ, Siegel IA (1951) Evaluation of the Rucker method of episiotomy repair as to perineal pain. *Am J Surg* **82**: 251–5

Myles MF (1971) *Textbook for Midwives*. 7th edn. Churchill Livingstone, London

Oboro VO, Tabowei TO, Loto OM, Bosah JO (2003) A multicentre evaluation of the two-layer repair of perineal trauma after birth. *J Obstet Gynaecol* **1**: 5–8

Olah KS (1994) Subcuticular perineal repair using a new continuous technique. *Br J Midwif* **2**(2): 67–71

Quick C, Thomas P (2000) *Principles of Surgical Management*. 1st edn. Oxford University Press, Oxford

Radcliffe W (1967) *Milestones in Midwifery*. John Wright and Sons Ltd, Bristol

Rhodes P (1995) *A Short History of Clinical Midwifery*. 1st edn. Books for Midwives Press, Cheshire

Rix JA (1992) Painful and perineal problem. *Daily Telegraph,* September: 14

Röckner G, Henningsson A, Wahlberg V, Olund A (1988) Evaluation of episiotomy and spontaneous tears of perineum during childbirth. *Scand J Caring Sci* **2**(1): 19–24

Rucker MP (1930) Perineorraphy with longitudinal sutures. *Virgina Medical Monthly*, July: 238–9

Scally G, Donaldson LJ (1998) Clinical governance and the drive for quality improvements in the new NHS in England. *Br Med J* **317**: 61–5

Silverton L (1993) *The Art and Science of Midwifery.* 1st edn. Prentice Hall, London

Sultan AH, Kamm MA, Hudson CN (1995) Obstetric perineal trauma: an audit of training. *J Obstet Gynaecol* **15**(1): 19–23

Taylor I, Karran SJ (1996) *Surgical Principles.* 1st edn. Oxford University Press, Oxford

Thacker SB, Banta HD (1983) Benefits and risks of episiotomy: an interpretive review of the English language literature 1860–1980. *Obstet Gynaecol Surv* **38**(6): 322–34

Tortora G, Grabowski S (1993) *Principles of Anatomy and Physiology.* 7th edn. Harper Collins College Publishers, New York

Towler J, Bramall J (1986) *Midwives in History and Society.* Croom Helm Ltd, Kent

Wood T (1999) Not suturing is safe. *The Practising Midwife* **2**(7): 15

# 5

## Episiotomy: the unkindest cut that persists

*Ian D Graham and Christine Davies*

Episiotomy is the surgical enlargement of the birth canal by an incision of the perineum at the time of birth (Thacker and Banta, 1983). There are two types, midline episiotomy (the incision is made in the midline) and mediolateral episiotomy (the incision begins in the midline but is directed laterally and downward away from the rectum) (Cunningham *et al*, 2001). The operation can be performed with a pair of scissors or a scalpel. Those who favour scissors maintain that they are less likely to damage the presenting part of the baby and more likely to promote homeostasis in the wound edges because of their crushing as well as cutting action. Those who favour the scalpel say that it minimizes trauma and is followed by better healing of the perineal wound (Enkin *et al*, 2004).

## Rationale for performing episiotomy

Historically, the use of episiotomy was advocated on the grounds that the operation (Carroli and Belizan, 2004; Cunningham *et al*, 2001; DeLee 1920; Eason and Feldman, 2000; Panter, 1980; Pomeroy, 1918; Shute, 1959):

- prevents severe perineal tears
- substitutes a straight, surgical cut for a ragged tear that might otherwise result
- is easier to repair and heals quicker than a tear
- is less painful postoperatively than a tear
- prevents pelvic relaxation and associated problems such as cystocele, rectocele and urinary incontinence
- improves sexual function of the woman and sexual satisfaction of her male partner
- reduces labour time
- reduces rates of asphyxia, cranial trauma, cerebral haemorrhage and mental retardation for the baby.

The suggested benefits of midline episiotomy are reported to be (Cunningham *et al*, 2001; Rageth *et al*, 1989):

- easy to repair
- rare incidence of faulty healing
- minimal pain
- excellent anatomical results
- less blood loss
- rarer incidence of dyspareunia.

The suggested benefit of mediolateral episiotomy is the minimized risk of extension of the incision (Bodner-Adler *et al*, 2001; Cunningham *et al*, 2001; Riskin-Mashiah *et al*, 2002), especially when forceps are used (Bodner-Adler *et al*, 2003).

## The questioning of routine episiotomy

The history of episiotomy is an interesting one as the operation became common practice without scientific evidence that it was beneficial. In the US, the routinization of episiotomy eventually resulted from strenuous lobbying efforts of a small group of obstetrician/gynecologists between 1915 and 1935. These physicians claimed that episiotomy prevented perineal lacerations, infant morbidity and mortality, and future gynaecological problems such as cystocele, rectocele, pelvic floor relaxation (Graham, 1997b). In England, the liberal use of episiotomy came about during the 1970s from pressure from obstetricians, although no overt campaigning for the practice occurred. In both places, routine episiotomy was encouraged by medical and extra medical factors which involved changes occurring in the dominant belief systems in obstetrics, maternity care practices, and the obstetric and midwifery professions (Graham, 1997b).

Beginning in the 1970s in the English speaking world, the use of episiotomy became increasing challenged within medicine (Anonymous, 1968; Brody and Thompson, 1981; Chalmers, 1975; House, 1981; Mehl, 1978; Morris, 1981; Ratner, 1978; Russell, 1982; Taylor, 1982; Thacker and Banta, 1983; Wagner, 1994; Zander, 1982) and midwifery (lay and professional) (Anderson, 1977; Kitzinger, 1979; Levett, 1974; Willmot, 1979) and by childbirth educators, organizations, the women's health movement, and childbearing women (Adamson, 1978; Anonymous, 1976; Boston Women's Health Collective, 1973; Bruce, 2001; Davis, 1976; Froshaug, 1974; Haire, 1972; Kitzinger, 1972; Kitzinger, 1981; Kitzinger and Walters, 1981; Yunker, 1975). This questioning created a climate conducive to submitting episiotomy to randomized clinical trials to determine the benefits of the routine use of the procedure. Six of these studies were published between 1984 and 1994 (Argentine Episiotomy Trial Collaborative Group 1993; Eltorkey *et al*, 1994; Harrison *et al*, 1984; House *et al*, 1986; Klein *et al*, 1992; Sleep *et al*, 1984). The results of a seventh trial have recently been published (Dannecker *et al*, 2004). The trials were undertaken in England (House *et al*, 1986; Sleep *et al*, 1984) Ireland (Harrison *et al*, 1984), Canada (Klein *et al*, 1992), Argentina (Argentine Episiotomy Trial Collaborative Group, 1993), Saudi Arabia (Eltorkey *et al*, 1994), and Germany (Dannecker *et al*, 2004). In addition, over the past twenty years a number of reviews of the literature have been published summarizing the evidence and supporting the restrictive use of episiotomy (Carroli and Belizan, 2004; David, 1993; Enkin *et al*, 1989; Fraser, 1983; Hirsch, 1997; House, 1981; Kolbl, 2001; Schlomer *et al*, 2003; Sleep *et al*, 1989; Smith *et al*, 1993; Thacker and Banta, 1983; Woolley, 1995a; Woolley, 1995b).

## The state of evidence for episiotomy

Carroli and Belizan have conducted the most recent systematic review of the randomized clinical trial literature using Cochrane Collaboration methodology to determine the possible benefits and risks of restrictive episiotomy versus routine episiotomy and the beneficial and detrimental effects of the use of midline episiotomy in comparison with mediolateral episiotomy (Carroli and Belizan, 2004). The review identified nine trials. The six trials designed to evaluate the benefits of episiotomy were included in the review (Argentine Episiotomy Trial Collaborative Group, 1993; Eltorkey *et al*, 1994; Harrison *et al*, 1984; House *et al*, 1986; Klein *et al*, 1992; Sleep *et al*, 1984; Sleep, 1987). Three trials that set out to evaluate the effectiveness of mediolateral versus midline episiotomy were excluded because of their poor methodological quality (Coats *et al*, 1980; Henriksen *et al*, 1992; Werner *et al*, 1991). Mediolateral episiotomy was the method of incision for all the trials except for the North American trial where midline episiotomy was performed (Klein *et al*, 1992). In total 4850 women participated in the six trials (2810 primipara and 2040 multipara women).

The review revealed that there is a lower risk of posterior perineal trauma (relative risk [RR] 0.88, 95% confidence interval [CI] 0.84 to 0.92), need for suturing perineal trauma (RR 0.74, 95% CI 0.71 to 0.77), and healing complications at seven days (RR 0.69, 95% CI 0.56 to 0.85) with the restrictive use of episiotomy. There is no difference in the incidence of major outcomes such as severe vaginal or perineal trauma, nor in pain, dyspareunia or urinary incontinence between the restrictive and routine/liberal use of episiotomy. The only disadvantage shown in the restrictive use of episiotomy is an increased risk of anterior perineal trauma (RR 1.79, 95% CI 1.55 to 2.07). Carroli and Belizan concluded that there is evidence to support the restrictive use of episiotomy compared to routine episiotomy (irrespective of the type of episiotomy performed). This finding applied to both primipara and multipara women. The results of this systematic review are also supported by the results of a recent RCT which compared the use of episiotomy only for fetal indications versus using episiotomy when a tear was presumed to be imminent (Dannecker *et al*, 2004). Because Carroli and Belizan excluded the three RCTs that focused specifically on the type of episiotomy, they concluded that there was insufficient evidence to indicate whether midline or mediolateral episiotomy is more beneficial. Many observational studies, however, have reported on the incidence of adverse effects associated with both midline and mediolateral episiotomy. In these studies, midline episiotomy is associated with an increased risk of third degree tears and anal incontinence (Eason *et al*, 2002; Helwig *et al*, 1993; Jander and Lyrenas, 2001; Klein *et al*, 1994; Labrecque *et al*, 1997; Shiono *et al*, 1990; Signorello *et al*, 2000). Mediolateral episiotomy is associated with lower pelvic floor functioning, dyspareunia and pain (Sartore *et al*, 2004). Thacker has recently called for a well-designed RCT comparing mediolateral and midline episiotomy to settle the issue once and for all (Thacker, 2000).

## Current policy and practice recommendations

Over the past fifteen years, the lack of evidence supporting the routine use of episiotomy has been disseminated and the international acceptance of this approach to perineal management can be seen in policy statements and clinical practice recommendations issued by many prominent public health and professional bodies. For example, the World Health Organization (WHO) recommends that episiotomy be used only for select indicators: complicated vaginal delivery (breech, shoulder dystocia, forceps, vacuum); scarring from female genital cutting or poorly healed third or fourth degree tears; fetal distress; insufficient progress of delivery; and threatened third degree tear (including third degree tear in a previous delivery) (WHO, 1996; WHO, 2000; WHO and PAHO, 1985). The Latin American Center for Perinatology and Human Development (CLAP) and the Pan American Health Organization (PAHO) recommend restrictive rather than routine use of episiotomy (CLAP, 2004). The Royal College of Obstetricians and Gynaecologists (RCOG) in the UK recommends that routine episiotomy be abandoned and a policy of restricting use of episiotomy to specific maternal and fetal indicators be adopted (Royal College of Obstetricians and Gynaecologists, 2000; Royal College of Obstetricians and Gynaecologists, 2002). The American College of Obstetricians and Gynecologists (ACOG) recommends that episiotomy be used to aid in the management of delivery in some situations, but states that routine use of the procedure is not necessary (American Academy of Pediatrics and American College of Obstetricians and Gynecologists, 1997). The American College of Nurse-Midwives (ACNM) recommends that episiotomy only be used to relieve fetal or maternal distress, or when the perineum is responsible for a lack of progress (American College of Nurse-Midwives, 2004). The Society of Obstetricians and Gynecologists of Canada (SOGC) recommends that episiotomy only be used to expedite delivery in the case of fetal compromise or maternal distress and lack of progress (Society of Obstetricians and Gynaecologists of Canada, 1998). The Federal Department of Health in Canada (Health Canada) also recommends that episiotomy only be used in the case of special fetal or maternal indications (Health Canada, 2000). Other organizations supporting the restrictive use of episiotomy are the Board on Global Health (BGH), a board of the US Institute of Medicine, a component of the US National Academy of Sciences (Board on Global Health and Institute of Medicine, 2003) and Maternal and Neonatal Health (MNH), a United States Agency for International Development (USAID) organization (MNH, 2004).

While there is generally a growing agreement about restricting the use of episiotomy, no such consensus has emerged as to what constitutes an appropriate episiotomy rate. Based on their RCT, Carroli and Belizan have indicated that a rate above 30% for primiparous women cannot be justified (Argentine Episiotomy Trial Collaborative Group, 1993). Some have suggested a rate of 20% is appropriate (Henriksen *et al*, 1992). Still others have suggested that it should be about 10% for primips and 5% for multips (Anonymous, 1994).

## The current use of episiotomy internationally

Episiotomy is a common obstetrical procedure, yet statistics on the use of operation are not always easily located. The haphazard way that national statistics on episiotomy are often collected and reported, if they happen to be collected and reported at all, is an indication of just how widely accepted the operation still is in many countries. It also indicates the lack of significance that has been placed on it by health officials. We have attempted to track down episiotomy rates from a number of countries. When truly national rates were not available or accessible we searched for studies which reported on the use of episiotomy in specific settings (eg. the use of episiotomy in one or several hospitals). Furthermore, despite the well known relationship between parity and the use of episiotomy (primiparous women having higher episiotomy rates), national episiotomy statistics by parity have not been systematically collected in many countries. Caution must be exercised when interpreting an episiotomy rate that is provided for the entire childbearing population, as this rate is influenced by the fertility rate and the resulting proportion of the population that is primiparous and multiparous (the episiotomy rate for primiparous women is usually higher than the rate for the total population).

*Table 5.1* presents episiotomy rates for the years 1995–2003 by selected regions and countries. *Figure 5.1* presents these data graphically to illustrate the considerable variation in the use of episiotomy. The episiotomy rates that include both primiparous and multiparous women range from as low as 9.7% (Sweden) to 100% (Taiwan). Rates for primiparous women range from 63.3% (South Africa) to 100% (Guatemala). Data from Eastern and Central Europe are limited although reports from the mid-1990s indicated that episiotomy was practiced routinely (90–100%) in this area of Europe (Chalmers, 1995; Wagner, 1994) (not included in *Table 5.1*, as these statistics are for the period prior to 1995). It is interesting to note some similarities in the episiotomy rate by language. For example, in English speaking countries the rate is on the lower side and ranges from 11% (Australia) to 32.7% (USA). In almost all Spanish speaking countries the primip rate is quite high ranging from 69.2% (Mexico) to 100% (Guatemala). The rate for Spain (87.3%) is more similar to the episiotomy rate found in South and Central America than it is to the rates of its European Union neighbours.

**Variation in episiotomy rates within countries**

Not only is there large variation in the use of episiotomy from country to country, there is often also variation within countries. The 2000–2001 episiotomy rate by Canadian provinces reveals that the use of the surgery ranges from 3% (Nunavut) to 31% (Quebec) (Health Canada, 2003). In the US, the episiotomy rate also varies from region to region. The highest rate in 2000 was in the Northeast, 38%, and the lowest was in the West, 27% (Kozak *et al*, 2002). In a study of five hospitals located in five non-contiguous states, Hueston found that the 1991–1992 episiotomy rate varied from 63 to 77% (Hueston, 1996). A similar observation has been made for hospitals in Ireland. Within Ireland, total episiotomy rates in 1998 varied between 7 and 47%. Primiparous rates varied between 13.3 and 80%, while multiparous rates varied between 2 and 40% (Cuidiu, 1999). A study of thirty-nine hospitals in the Netherlands found the 1995 episiotomy rate varied from 7.6% to 42.1% in spontaneous term deliveries (Heres *et al*, 1995). In Argentina, the total episiotomy rate for 1995 was found to range between 33% and 62.5% in different hospitals (Cravchik *et al*, 1998). In England, there is little variation in episiotomy rate by region. National statistics for 2002–2003 reveal the rate by region differed by only 3%. However, only a decade earlier, Williams *et al* in their cross-sectional survey of 100 NHS hospitals found the episiotomy rate varied appreciably throughout the regions and hospitals in the UK, from 26% to 67% (Williams *et al*, 1998). Variation in episiotomy rates by hospital in Sweden has been observed by Rockner *et al* in 1989 and 1995, although the variation was less in 1995 (Rockner and Fianu-Jonasson, 1999; Rockner and Olund, 1991). A 1999 observational study of four hospitals in Shanghai, China, revealed that the episiotomy rate ranged from 65% to 93% (Qian *et al*, 2001).

## Table 5.1: Selected episiotomy rates by region and country

| Region | Country | Year | Primiparous | Total |
|---|---|---|---|---|
| North America | Canada[1] | 2000–2001 | | 23.8 |
| | USA[2] | 2000 | | 32.7 |
| Central and South America | Argentina[3; 4] | 1995–1998, 1996 | 85.7 | 28.5 |
| | Mexico[4] | 1995–1998 | 69.2 | |
| | Panama[4] | 1995–1998 | 81.8 | |
| | Colombia[4] | 1995–1998 | 86.2 | |
| | Nicaragua[4] | 1995–1998 | 86.3 | |
| | Bolivia[4] | 1995–1998 | 90.8 | |
| | Paraguay[4] | 1995–1998 | 91.5 | |
| | Honduras[4] | 1995–1998 | 92 | |
| | Brazil[4] | 1995–1998 | 94.2 | |
| | Peru[4] | 1995–1998 | 94.4 | |
| | Dominican Republic[4] | 1995–1998 | 94.9 | |
| | Uruguay[4] | 1995–1998 | 95.1 | |
| | Chile[4] | 1995–1998 | 95.9 | |
| | Ecuador[4] | 1995–1998 | 96.2 | |
| | Guatemala[5] | 2001 | 100 (estimate) | |
| Northern Europe | Sweden[6] | 1992–2000 | 24.5 | 9.7 |
| | Denmark[7] | 2002–2003 | | 12 |
| | Finland[8] | 2002 | | 36.2 |
| Western Europe | England[9] | 2002–2003 | | 13 |
| | Scotland[7] | 2002–2003 | | 16.3 |
| | Netherlands[10] | 1995 | | 24.5 |
| | Germany[7] | 2002–2003 | | 44.4 |
| | Switzerland[11] | 2004 | | 46 |
| | Ireland[6] | 1999–2000 | | 46 |
| | France[7; 12] | 2002–2003 | 71.3 | 49.5 |
| | Italy[6] | 1999 | | 58 |
| | Turkey[13] | 1999–2000 | | 64 |
| | Spain[14] | 1995 | | 87.3 |
| Eastern Europe | Bulgaria[15; 16] | 1996, 1997 | 77.1 | 45.6 |
| | Russia[17] | 1997 | | 46.2 |
| Asia | Nepal[18] | 2003 | 37 | 42.9–67.3 |
| | China[19] | 2001 | | 82 |
| | Taiwan[20] | 2002 | | 100 (estimate) |
| Middle East | Israel[21] | 2001 | | 37.6 |
| Oceania | New Zealand[22] | 2001 | | 11 |
| | Australia[23; 24] | 1996–19997, 2000 | | 12.8 |
| Africa | Burkina Faso[25] | 1998 | 37 | 14 |
| | Nigeria[26] | 2001 | | 20 |
| | Botswana[27] | 1998–2000 | | 20.7 |
| | Zimbabwe[28] | 1997–1998 | | 27 |
| | South Africa[29] | 2003 | | 63.3–67.5 |

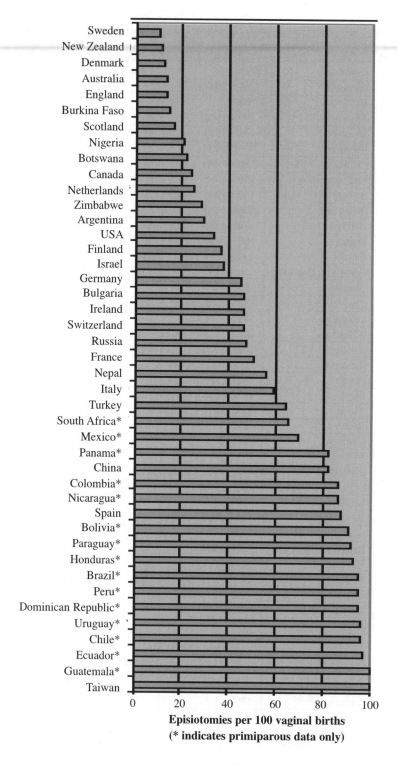

**Figure 5.1: Graphical presentation of recent episiotomy rates by country, 1995–2003**

## Variation in episiotomy rates within the same professional group

Not only can episiotomy rates vary between and within countries, they can vary considerably within the same provider group in the same institution. In one study of twenty experienced labour ward midwives in Dublin, episiotomy rates by individual caregiver ranged from a low of 6% to a high of 84% (Begley, 2002). Similarly in England, Wilkerson studied twenty-one midwives in one hospital and observed huge variations between midwives and concluded that the variation suggested episiotomy was determined not by the condition of the mother or baby but by which provider was allocated to the case (Wilkerson, 1984). In an observational study of thirty midwives in Denmark, Henriksen *et al* (1994) found that the rate of episiotomies performed varied from less than 10% to over 70%.

This brief and selected review of episiotomy rates revealed considerable variation in the use of the operation by country, within country, and within the same professional group. These differences are not likely to be well explained by differences in the childbearing population. This finding suggests that the use of the operation may not be guided solely by clinical indications or by practice guidelines about the procedure. What then explains the considerable variation in the use of episiotomy?

## Factors associated with the use of episiotomy

A number of clinical and maternal factors have been shown to be associated with the use of episiotomy in several observational studies. Well known risk factors for episiotomy are:

- instrumental delivery (forceps or vacuum extraction) (Dimitrov *et al*, 1997; Goldberg *et al*, 2002; Howden *et al*, 2004; Hueston, 1996; Rockner and Fianu-Jonasson, 1999; Shorten and Shorten, 2000)
- low parity (Dimitrov *et al*, 1997; Howden *et al*, 2004; Hueston 1996; Shorten and Shorten, 2000; Zondervan *et al*, 1995)
- epidural anaesthesia (Hueston, 1996; Newman *et al*, 2001; Robinson *et al*, 2001; Rockner and Fianu-Jonasson, 1999; Shorten and Shorten, 2000)
- duration of second stage (Hueston, 1996; Robinson *et al*, 2001; Williams *et al*, 1998; Zondervan *et al*, 1995)
- birthweight (Dimitrov *et al*, 1997; Howden *et al*, 2004; Shorten and Shorten, 2000)
- fetal macrosomia (Hueston, 1996; Robinson *et al*, 2001)
- younger maternal age (Howden *et al*, 2004; Weber and Meyn, 2002)
- history of Caesarean section (Howden *et al*, 2004)
- premature birth (Dimitrov *et al*, 1997).

Interestingly, a number of non-clinical factors have also been shown or suggested to be incidentally related to episiotomy use. These include the category or type of maternity care provider, site of care, model of care delivery, and the race, ethnicity and social class of the parturient. In many studies, the relationship between these factors and episiotomy persists even after controlling for clinical and maternal factors.

## Category of maternity care provider

A fairly consistent finding throughout the world is that consultant obstetricians are the group that make the most use of episiotomy. Family physicians use the operation less than obstetricians but more than midwives. While professional midwives tend to be low users of the procedure, lay midwives or traditional birth attendants have even lower episiotomy rates than their professional counterparts. For example, over a decade ago, a survey of obstetric practitioners in New Mexico revealed that the use of episiotomy was least frequent among lay midwives (93% responded that they performed episiotomy for less than one fourth of primiparas), more frequent among nurse-midwives (24% performed episiotomy one more than three quarters of primiparas), more frequent again by family physicians (64% performed episiotomies on more than three quarters of primiparas), more frequent again by obstetricians (81% performed episiotomies on more than three quarters of primiparas) and most frequently used by obstetric residents (100% performed episiotomies on more than three quarters of primiparas) (Graham *et al*, 1990). Hueston (1996) conducted a retrospective review of 8647 births (6458 vaginal births) during 1991 and 1992 at five medical centres in the US and found that the episiotomy rate was 73% for obstetricians, 58% for family physicians, and 38% for nurse-midwives. This finding remained after controlling for parity and instrumental delivery. Another review of 1576 consecutive term, singleton, spontaneous vaginal births at Brigham and Women's Hospital in Boston between 1 December, 1994 and 31 July, 1996 found that the episiotomy rate was 56% for physicians in private practice attending women at the hospital, 33% for faculty obstetricians, and 21% for midwives. Again, this finding persisted after controlling for other possible confounding factors (Robinson *et al*, 2000). Other studies have also observed that obstetricians used episiotomy more often than midwives, even when the medical conditions of the women being attended by the practitioners were taken into account (Anonymous, 1993; Gerrits *et al*, 1994; Hundley *et al*, 1994; Kaufman and MacDonald, 1988). A similar finding was reported by a 1990 Canadian study evaluating the implementation of a pilot nurse-midwifery programme which found that the episiotomy rates were lower in women served by midwives (16%), and higher in women served by physicians (33%) (Harvey *et al*, 1996). In Australia, Shorten and Shorten conducted a retrospective study of 2028 Australian women delivering vaginally and concluded that the difference in episiotomy rates between private (36%) and public (26%) care reflected the difference between physician and midwife-led care (Shorten and Shorten, 2000). In the Netherlands, an observational study using the Dutch National Obstetric Database of 1990 revealed that that gynaecologists performed more episiotomies than midwives (Zondervan *et al*, 1995).

A multicentre study in Burkina Faso in Africa revealed that the episiotomy rate for registered midwives was 46% for primiparas and 10% for multiparas compared with 26% and 4% for auxiliary midwives practicing in rural areas (Lorenz *et al*, 1998). Even among traditional birth attendants (TBA), one study of 127 TBAs in Brazil revealed that the episiotomy rate differed by how the attendant learned to attend births. The episiotomy rate of TBAs who had learned at hospital was 17% compared to 15% for those who had learned by themselves and 3% for those who had learned from another TBA (Carvalho *et al*, 1998). A Nigerian study revealed that TBAs in a rural area did not practice episiotomies, while Western-trained nurse-midwives and physicians made use of the procedure (Brink, 1982). In a retrospective study of 27,702 women who gave birth between 1995 and 2000 in one large urban academic hospital in the US, the strongest predictor of episiotomy was care by a private practitioner even when controlling for fetal and maternal characteristics (Howden *et al*, 2004). The overall episiotomy rate was 57% for private practitioners and 12% for academic practitioners (midwives, faculty and residents).

Not only is the use of episiotomy related to category of obstetric provider, so is the style of the incision. A prospective survey of fifty physicians and seventy-eight midwives from a large tertiary referral obstetric hospital and obstetrics department of a district general hospital in the UK, asked respondents to draw how they perform an episiotomy. The pictorial questionnaire revealed that physicians and midwives make different styles of incisions: physicians' incisions are longer and have larger angles (Tincello *et al*, 2003).

## Site of care

In addition to category of provider, Hueston's study also found that site of care (data were captured on births at five centres) was independently associated with episiotomy (the episiotomy rate ranged from 39%–78%) (Hueston, 1996). In a national survey of 542 Canadian hospitals (91% response rate, n=523 hospitals), Kaczorowski *et al* (1998) found that university-affiliated hospitals and non-teaching hospitals were more likely than university teaching hospitals to have episiotomy rates over 40% for primiparous women. They also found that large hospitals were more likely than small hospitals to have episiotomy rates over 20% for multiparous women (Kaczorowski *et al*, 1998). In a survey of 988 women delivering at either a consult-led maternity unit or a hospital birthing centre in Nepal, Rana *et al* (2003) found that women delivering at the midwife-led hospital birthing centre were less likely to undergo an episiotomy than women at the consultant-led maternity unit. Zondervan *et al*'s (1995) observational study in the Netherlands found that episiotomy rates were lower in university hospitals than in large, non-university hospitals. In a retrospective comparison of free-standing birth centres versus hospitals in Berlin (4,072 births in total), birth centres were found to have higher episiotomy rates for both primiparas and multiparas (David *et al*, 1999).

Given the relationship between provider category and use of episiotomy and that certain categories of providers may be associated with specific locations (eg. obstetricians with hospitals), it is not surprising that studies have also shown that location of care can be related to the incidence of episiotomy.

## Continuity of care

Some studies have examined the relationship between the model of maternity care provided and woman's likelihood of receiving an episiotomy. A prospective comparative study of 728 English women receiving one-to-one midwifery care (high continuity of care) versus 675 women receiving conventional care found that lower episiotomy rates were achieved in the group with the higher continuity of care (OR 0.70, 95%CI (0.5, 0.98)) (Page *et al*, 1999). A UK randomized controlled trial of the efficacy of midwife-managed care versus shared care (care divided among midwives, hospital doctors and general practitioners) found that midwife managed care generated less episiotomies than shared care (Turnbull *et al*, 1996). A 1999 Cochrane Systematic Review of two randomized controlled trials (Flint *et al*, 1989; Rowley *et al*, 1995) found that women receiving continuity of care from the same midwives or small midwifery group were less likely to be given an episiotomy (OR 0.75, 95% CI [0.60 to 0.94]) (Hodnett, 1999).

## Race, ethnicity and class

Studies of multi-ethnic countries or communities have found that a woman's race can affect her likelihood of receiving an episiotomy. Most studies have found that minority women are less likely to receive an episiotomy, although this is not always the case.

In the US, four studies have reported that white women were more likely to be given an episiotomy than black women, even when controlling for age, parity, insurance status and operative vaginal delivery (Goldberg *et al*, 2002; Howard *et al*, 2000; Weber and Meyn, 2002; Weeks and Kozak, 2001). A UK cross-sectional survey of 101 randomly-selected NHS hospitals (forty consecutive, low-risk primiparae from each hospital) found that non-white women were more likely to be given an episiotomy, with women from the Indian sub-continent and the Orient almost twice and five times more likely to receive an episiotomy respectively (Williams *et al*, 1998). Data from Australia (The New South Wales Midwives Data Collection, Epidemiology and Surveillance Branch, NSW Health Department), showed that aboriginal mothers were less likely to receive an episiotomy than non-aboriginal mothers (NSW Health Department, 1997).

Relationships between race and ethnicity have also been observed in other European and Latin American countries. An Italian study of the mode of delivery of 13,945 women at one hospital over a period of ten years, found that women of non-EU origin were less likely to be given an episiotomy (Diani *et al*, 2003). The Zondervan observational study using the Dutch National Obstetric Database of 1990 (containing records for 65,313 women), found that, independent of known risk factors for episiotomy, Mediterranean, Hindu and Creole women were less likely to have an episiotomy than Dutch women (Zondervan *et al*, 1995). In a Brazilian birth cohort study involving 5,305 children, African Brazilian (black) women were found to be 30% less likely to undergo an episiotomy than white women (Barros *et al*, 2001).

Several studies have examined whether a woman's class (often inferred through her use of public versus private health care) affects her likelihood of episiotomy. These studies have found that private health care is an important predictor of episiotomy use. In the US, Goldberg conducted an electronic audit of the medical procedures database at Thomas Jefferson University Hospital over the period 1983–2000 (34,048 women) and found that Medicaid insurance (ie. being poor) was associated with a decreased incidence of episiotomy (Goldberg *et al*, 2002). Similar findings have been reported using the US National Hospital Discharge Survey (Weber and Meyn, 2002; Weeks and Kozak, 2001). In Australia, Shorten and Shorten found that privately-insured women were twice as likely as publicly-insured women to undergo an episiotomy (Shorten and Shorten, 2000). In Brazil, Diniz and Chacham have argued that class is an important predictor of episiotomy because wealthier women (using the private healthcare system) are more likely to opt out of vaginal birth altogether and have a Caesarean section, while women using the public system are more likely to deliver vaginally and receive an episiotomy (Diniz and Chacham, 2004).

## Some sociological thoughts on the role of beliefs and attitudes and the use of episiotomy

A sociological analysis of the considerable variation in the use of episiotomy by country, within countries, between and among obstetric provider category in the same country, and the relationship of the operation to non-clinical factors, such as race and class would suggest that individual providers' attitudes and beliefs towards episiotomy, birth more generally, and women are likely at play. The obvious explanation is that differences between provider categories can be attributed to differences in training received by obstetricians, family physicians, midwives, and traditional birth attendants. While this is true, it begs a question about why the training and professional socialization is different and what are the differences in world views and paradigms between the groups with respect to their beliefs about the nature of the perineum, episiotomy and birth that are instilled during their training.

In a unique study, following the completion of a randomized controlled trial of episiotomy, Klein *et al* surveyed the forty-three participating physicians who attended 447 births about their beliefs in the putative benefits of episiotomy (Klein *et al*, 1995). They then divided the physicians into quartiles based on the strength of the views that they held about episiotomy: very favourable, favourable, unfavourable, or very unfavourable. They then undertook a post-hoc analysis of the trial data and compared use of obstetric practices and subsequent patient outcomes of each of these groups of clinicians. Although characteristics of the women attended by each category of physician were similar (eg. in terms of parity, age, height, weight gain, baby's birth weight), doctors with more favourable views of episiotomy were more like to perform episiotomy. Furthermore, women attended by these physicians received more oxytocin augmentations of labour and had shorter labours than women attended by physicians with unfavourable views of episiotomy. Klein *et al* concluded that physicians with more favourable views of episiotomy were more likely to consider apparently normal labour as abnormal and in keeping with this perspective, were also more likely to intervene in the birth process and use techniques to expedite labour. Using the same questionnaire, Labrecque *et al* analyzed 5,419 primiparous singleton vaginal births attended by sixteen physicians between 1985 and 1993 and found that physicians' beliefs about the value of episiotomy were related to use of the procedure (Labrecque *et al*, 1997). Physicians who did not believe that episiotomy was associated with third and fourth degree tears were more likely to perform the surgery.

This conclusion is also supported by a cross-country socio-historical analysis of episiotomy (Graham, 1996; Graham, 1997; Graham, 1998). In both the US and UK, the routine use of episiotomy that occurred during the twentieth century came about only after a radical shift in the obstetric belief systems of both countries. In the USA, the routine use of episiotomy, which became popular beginning in the late 1930s, did so after obstetricians succeeded in recasting birth from a normal process that was thought to require very little intervention to a more pathological process that was believed to necessitate prophylactic intervention to diminish or prevent fetal and maternal damage. In the UK, the shift that removed some of the longstanding barriers to the more liberal use of episiotomy was the acceptance of 'active management of labour' during the 1970s, the underlying principle being the superiority of obstetric intervention over physiologic processes. Once birth was seen in more pathological terms, then acceptance of the putative prophylactic benefits of episiotomy supported its widespread use. In keeping with the episiotomy statistics, the history and literature of episiotomy also reveals that provider groups do not always possess the same beliefs, and that competing belief systems can encourage and support change by offering philosophical justification for challenging existing practices. This has been the case with the questioning of the liberal use of episiotomy by midwives and general and family medicine practitioners on both sides of the Atlantic. These groups' belief in birth as an essentially physiological process not requiring routine surgical intervention has been central to their challenging of episiotomy and their lower use of episiotomy for low risk women than obstetricians.

Very much linked to beliefs systems about the nature of childbirth and the superiority of intervention is the phenomenon referred to as the medicalization of childbirth (hospitalization, use of interventions, etc). A number of observers have argued that medicalization of childbirth in less developed countries has supported the use of episiotomy. In an article on an education program for maternity care providers in St Petersburg, Russia, Chalmers wrote that:

> *Birth conditions and procedures in the former Soviet Union... are characterized by a traditional, obstetric intervention, physician-directed model. Practices such as... episiotomies... are almost routine.*
>
> (Chalmers *et al*, 1998)

In a letter to the *British Medical Journal*, Yeh wrote of the situation in Taiwan:

> *Alas, in childbirth, medicalization has taken hold throughout the obstetric profession. Nearly every intervention in childbirth is perceived as necessary and good... All women in labour undergo routine midline episiotomy. Every woman is subjected to this regardless of gestation (term or preterm). The episiotomy rate approaches 100%.*
>
> (Yeh, 2002)

In an article on rates of unnecessary obstetric procedures in Sao Paulo, Diniz wrote that:

> *In the last fifty years, a rapid increase in the use of technology to start, augment, accelerate, regulate and monitor the process of birth has frequently led to the adoption of inadequate, unnecessary and sometimes dangerous interventions... The 94.2% rate of episiotomy... In most medical schools in Brazil, providers are still taught the intervention model. Surgical ability and sophisticated pathology are highly valued, while comparatively little attention is paid to women-centred care for normal deliveries, and good communication and interaction with all birthing women.*
>
> (Diniz and Chacham, 2004)

The case has also been made that the previously high reliance on episiotomy in the US was imported into other countries and cultures with little questioning as obstetric intervention undertaken in the US was perceived as being more progressive or superior to more traditional approaches of restricting the use of episiotomy (Kitzinger, 1979; Lorenz *et al*, 1998).

Other attitudes that have been suggested to influence the use of episiotomy have to do with misogyny and the understanding of women and their bodies as passive or non-human. Kitzinger describes how obstetric language constructs women's bodies as passive using phrases such as 'lazy uterus', and non-human, using phrases such as 'pubic arch' and 'pelvic floor'. She suggests that the linking of the female anatomy with a passive, unliving world facilitates the decision to perform obstetric interventions (Kitzinger, 1999). Diniz and colleagues have made a similar observation:

*If they believe the vulva and vagina are passive, it is difficult even for them to understand these tissues are able to distend for birth and contract afterwards. Thus, through episiotomy, physicians deconstruct and reconstruct the vagina, in accordance with cultural beliefs.*

(Diniz and Chacham, 2004)

Stotland argues that interventions affecting perfectly normal female functioning such as episiotomy 'can be attributed to men's unconscious (and conscious) curiosity, jealousy, hostility, and helplessness about female reproduction, coupled with the fact that men have dominated the field of medicine for most of its history' (Stotland, 2004). Davis-Floyd, an American anthropologist, has also argued that the demise of the midwife and the rise of the male-attended, mechanically manipulated birth followed close on the heels of the wide cultural acceptance of the metaphor of the body-as-machine in the West and the accompanying acceptance of the metaphor of the female body as a defective machine — a metaphor which eventually formed the philosophical foundation of modern obstetrics. Obstetrics was thus challenged from its beginnings to develop tools and technologies for the manipulation and improvement of the inherently defective and therefore anomalous and dangerous process of birth (Davis-Floyd, 1990).

A biological explanation for the variation in episiotomy use by racial and ethnic groups might be genetic differences between the groups. A sociological explanation might be that maternity care providers believe that different racial/ethnic groups have different risks of severe laceration (Manzer, 2002) which results in providers differentially using episiotomy in the hopes of minimizing these risks. The belief that women's level of civilization (ie. race) or social standing affected her risk of perineal damage was not uncommon early in the last century and is illustrated in the following quotation from a prominent US obstetrician:

*Labour should be a physiological and natural process, and it seems strange at first sight that such a process is so often associated with serious damage to the woman. But this is the price civilized women pay for her elevation from the original savage state, and the higher or more artificial the civilization, the dearer the cost. It has been seen by many army surgeons, that Indian squaws on the plains are very rarely injured in this way, for with their strong muscles and elastic tissues, and with the smaller fetal head that is the sign of lesser mental development of the race, the maternal soft parts are subjected to nothing like the stain that is put on them in the case of women bred in towns, ill-developed physically, and bearing children*

> *that spring from a long succession of brain workers, and whose heads are*
> *extraordinarily large in comparison with their bodies.*

(Hirst, 1902)

More research is needed to explore racial and class differences in episiotomy and the influence providers' beliefs have on obstetric practice.


## Knowledge, transfer and reducing inappropriate use of episiotomy

Statistics on episiotomy reveal that the use of the procedure can change. *Figure 5.2* presents the longitudinal data we were able to locate on the use of episiotomy for the UK, USA, Canada and Australia since 1970. In all these English speaking countries there has been a steady decline in the use of the procedure, although the slope of the decline differs between countries. Although few data are available prior to 1980, it appears that the use of the procedure began declining around 1980 before the release of the results of the first episiotomy RCT (Graham, 1997b). Between 1980 and 2000 the relative decline in the use of episiotomy was 50% in the USA, 65% in Canada and 73% in England. Declining use of the procedure has also been reported in Europe. A Swedish study of sixty-two labour wards and a university hospital between 1989 and 1995 revealed a significant decrease in the use of episiotomy (a 34% decline in the procedure) (Rockner and Fianu-Jonasson, 1999). A study of birth methods at one Swiss clinic between 1986 and 1997 with over 344,328 births saw the episiotomy rate drop from 80% to lower than 15% (Eberhard and Geissbuehler, 2000).

### Strategies for reducing the use of episiotomy

In health care, it has historically been assumed that publication of research findings automatically lead to changes in practice. Unfortunately, one of the most consistent findings in health services research is that the transfer of research findings into practice is often unpredictable and can be a slow and haphazard process (Agency for Health Research and Quality, 2001). In the case of episiotomy, there has been considerable continuous declining use of the procedure during the past two decades in the English speaking world with relatively little intervention. Given *Figure 5.2*, it does not appear that the publication of the results of any one episiotomy RCT or systematic review can be attributed with producing a large precipitous decline in episiotomy. The diffusion of this growing body of evidence has, however, been very important in causing maternity care providers to re-evaluate their beliefs about the putative benefits of the operation (Marcus, 2004). Had this evidence not challenged providers' beliefs, there would have been less stimulus to restrict their use of the practice. Unfortunately, the evidence about episiotomy has not consistently been transferred to providers in all countries, especially developing ones. For example, Richards notes that there is generally a lack of awareness of Cochrane reviews in developing countries (Richards, 2004). In Zimbabwe it has been observed that midwives are less exposed to findings from systematic reviews and hold more traditional beliefs (Smith *et al*, 1999). In Brazil, the most used obstetrics textbook still supports the liberal use of episiotomy (Diniz and Chacham, 2004). An important precondition for reducing the use of episiotomy will be to ensure the transfer of the evidence about episiotomy into the knowledge base of indigenous and local providers in all countries.

Engaging healthcare providers in randomized controlled trials (and studies using other designs) is another strategy for promoting the rethinking of the use of episiotomy and reducing its use. In each of the episiotomy RCTs to date, the investigators were successful in reducing the use of episiotomy in the intervention arm. Additionally, Belizan and Carroli tracked the episiotomy rates of one hospital in Rosario Argentina before, during and after their randomized controlled trial (data from 1990–1996) (Belizan and Carroli, 1998). They found that after the randomized controlled trial, the total episiotomy rate dropped from 47.9% in 1990 to 28.5% in 1996. The 1996 rate was lower than the 30.1% rate achieved in the restrictive arm of the randomized controlled trial. Primiparous rates dropped from 92.9% in 1990 to 65.3% in 1996, a 26.9% drop. These data suggest that reductions in the use of episiotomy resulting from participation in an episiotomy trial may be sustained over time.

There have also been a number of active interventions to bring about the restrictive use of episiotomy. Most have not been rigorously evaluated to determine their effectiveness. The studies that have been conducted on the effectiveness of the strategies have tended to use pre-post study designs which are more susceptible to bias than experimental designs.

One of the first prospective observational studies specifically designed to lower the use of episiotomy was conducted by Henriksen *et al* in Denmark (Henriksen *et al*, 1994). The study involved recording the use of episiotomy by thirty midwives for a period of ten months and then providing each midwife with a graphical presentation of her own and colleagues episiotomy rates. The use of episiotomy in 3913 births was then monitored for the next nineteen months. The evaluation of the use of feedback and graphical profiles of rates of episiotomy revealed an absolute decline of 6.6% or a relative decline of 18% (the rate decreased from 37.1% to 30.5%) during the second time period that persisted until the end of the study. The feedback did not coincide with introduction of new guidelines regarding the use of episiotomy nor educational sessions, although the individual feedback did lead to some discussions about the practice among the midwives. Others have also reported positive experiences in the UK using the strategy of auditing midwifery use of episiotomy and reflecting this information back (Begley, 2002; Stratton *et al*, 1995) but Stratton *et al* suggested that continuous feedback is probably necessary to maintain the restrictive use of episiotomy (Stratton *et al*, 1995). Strictly speaking, the following strategy does not fall under the category of audit and feedback since it only involved implementing a labour chart that included a tick off box for whether an episiotomy was performed. However, this allowed the collection of data on the use of episiotomy that was used to stimulate discussion and professional communication about the practice. Lorenzo *et al* introduced the labour chart four to six months prior to the study in two urban and sixteen rural health facilities. Although no statistics were provided on the pre-post episiotomy rate, the researchers concluded that the introduction of the labour chart was a useful vehicle for changing professional behaviour (Lorenz *et al*, 1998).

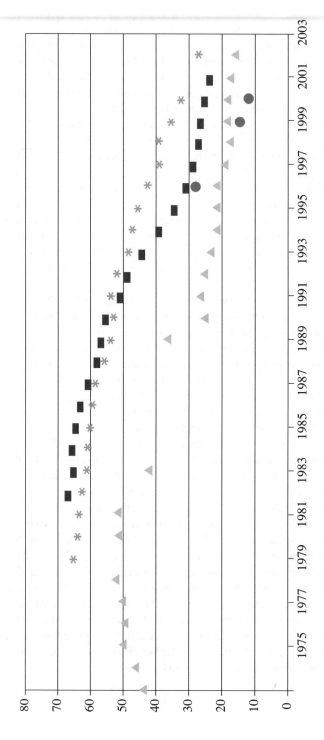

Figure 5.2: Episiotomy rates for English-speaking countries (Shorten and Shorten, 2000; Australian Institute of Health and Welfare and National Perinatal Statistics Unit, 2001; Australian Institute of Health and Welfare and National Perinatal Statistics Unit, 2003; Graham and Fowler-Graham, 1997a; Health Canada, 2003; England and Government Statistical Service, 2004; Goldberg et al, 2002; Kozak et al, 2002; Declerq et al, 2002; Weeks and Kozak, 2001; Robinson et al, 2000)

Reynolds conducted a before-and-after study which used a continuous quality improvement (CQI) program to reduce the use of episiotomy in one hospital in Canada (Reynolds, 1995). This study involved applying educational strategies to promote better understanding of what constitutes an appropriate episiotomy and true fetal distress as well as suggesting ways to reduce maternal exhaustion and manoeuvres to protect the perineum during childbirth. By the end of the study period (one year), the overall episiotomy rate declined from 44.5% to 33.3%. Bourget and Ymayo in Brazil have also had good success using a program of quality and continuous education which involved monthly educational seminars and workshops, training in emergency situations, and feedback to providers of their episiotomy rate. The study took place during an eight-month period (May–December, 1999) in one hospital in Sao Paulo with 4,000 births. The use of episiotomy declined from 90–100% to 18–22% (Bourget and Ymayo, 2000).

The largest and most well developed study to evaluate interventions to change the use of episiotomy is currently ongoing in South America. The study is a cluster randomized controlled trial of a behavioural intervention to increase the use of restrictive episiotomy and active management of the third stage of labour. The trial is taking place in Argentina and Uruguay and will involve twenty-four hospitals. At the twelve intervention hospitals, opinion leaders will be identified and trained in how to develop evidence-based guidelines which they will disseminate using a multifaceted approach involving seminars, academic detailing, reminders, and feedback of utilization rates. The control hospitals will continue to use their standard in-service training activities. Enrolment began in July 2003 with the completion date expected to be March 2006 (US National Library of Medicine, 2004).

A number of other strategies for reducing the use of episiotomy have also been undertaken or suggested although not evaluated in a rigorous way. For example, clinical skills training has been used in Guatemala to foster new maternal and neonatal practices and attitudes among nurses and doctors (MNH, 2004). Following the training, the participants reported favouring the restrictive use of episiotomy. Similarly, twelve workshops in evidence-based antenatal and intrapartum care were conducted in St Petersburg, Russia for health professionals. Following the workshops, more family-centred care was introduced, and a small reduction in the use of episiotomy was seen (49% to 46%) (Chalmers *et al*, 1998). The Better Births Initiative aims to introduce evidence-based maternal care to developing countries and improve women's experience of birth. In the South Africa pilot study, educational materials (posters, videos, booklets) were distributed, a workshop was conducted, and caregivers underwent a 'self-audit'. Episiotomy rates decreased after these initiatives (Smith *et al*, 2001). The Latin American Centre for Perinatology and Human Development (CLAP), Pan American Health Organization (PAHO) and the World Health Organization (WHO) are creating a program to promote evidence-based care and maternal outcomes in Latin America. Episiotomy is targeted as a practice that is not beneficial and is potentially harmful. An award will be given to hospitals meeting specific health indexes. Training packages and clinical guidelines will be provided to hospitals. Staff will also be trained to identify new medical evidence as it becomes available so as to improve continuously practices (CLAP, 2004).

Because midwives and traditional birth attendants often have lower rates of episiotomy, it is thought that promoting or empowering these caregivers could lead to a decrease in national episiotomy rates. A Brazilian study, which was transformed into a series of recommendations to the federal, state and municipal governments, made suggestions on how to empower existing traditional birth attendants, incorporate them into existing healthcare systems and practices, and increase the number of birth attendants through schools (Carvalho *et al*, 1998). A similar argument has also been put forth in the West. It has been suggested that establishing practice committees and promoting interdisciplinary clinical exchanges of information about evidence-based practice and techniques among nurses, nurse-midwives and obstetricians would provide an opportunity for greater cross-fertilization and result in the more evidence-based practice and restrictive use of episiotomy (Low *et al*, 2000; Simpson and Knox, 1999). An interdisciplinary approach to the issue of episiotomy is likely to be helpful in breaking down professional silos and facilitating the exchange of skills and perspectives which might be particularly important for obstetricians who may have less training and experience with non-interventionist approaches to childbirth.

One other strategy that contributed to the decline in the use of episiotomy in the UK and US was challenging of the practice by childbearing women, childbirth organizations and childbirth educators (Graham, 1997b). Magazine articles and websites continue to coach women on 'How to avoid an episiotomy' (Bruce, 2001; Griffin, 1995; Maier, 2000). Encouraging women to question their care and express their preferences is another strategy that could be used to change professional behaviour. This strategy, however, will be less effective in areas where rates of literacy and access to education and various forms of media are more limited.

## Conclusions

When used as a procedure of last resort, episiotomy has an important role to play in midwifery practice. Unfortunately in many countries, the routine use of episiotomy has often become accepted practice based solely on beliefs about the putative benefits of the procedure. Research from randomized controlled trials conducted over the past twenty years has consistently failed to support the liberal use of episiotomy. These studies have found that the restrictive use of episiotomy results in lower posterior perineal trauma, need for suturing perineal trauma, and healing complications with no differences in the incidence of major outcomes, such as severe vaginal or perineal trauma, pain, dyspareunia or urinary incontinence. These data provide the foundation for many national and international evidence-based practice recommendations that advocate the abandonment of routine episiotomy.

Despite the strong evidence that routine episiotomy is not beneficial (even harmful) and international clinical recommendations that it should be abandoned, the surgery is still being routinely performed in many parts of the world. Our review of the literature suggests that the continued reliance on episiotomy is largely supported by health care providers' beliefs about the operation and the nature of childbirth rather than the evidence. Bringing about reductions in the use of episiotomy will require ensuring that all providers are aware of the evidence supporting the restrictive use of episiotomy. This will involve making sure that the evidence about episiotomy is available in every language and targeted to all provider groups. It will also involve convincing providers to abandon their longstanding beliefs in the putative benefits of routine episiotomy. Beliefs can be quite resistant to change and take time to change. While the experience in the English speaking world was that the accumulation of evidence supporting the restricted use of episiotomy, coupled with advocacy efforts appear to have been sufficient to convince providers to limit their use of episiotomy, this has taken two decades. Developing and using interventions to transfer this knowledge should hasten the process. While limited, there is some data on the effectiveness of some interventions in reducing the use of episiotomy. Finally, it is essential that these providers be taught the skills to manage births without resorting to the incision (the focus of other chapters). This is particularly important as clinical experiences can reinforce (or overturn) one's beliefs about the value of one's actions. While changing professional behaviour is complex and can take a long time, the challenge now is to be persistent and find innovative ways of transferring the evidence about episiotomy into practice everywhere.

# References

Adamson L (1978) Unkind Cuts. *The Guardian* 11 January, 1978: 9

Agency for Health Research and Quality (2001) *Translating Research Into Practice* (TRIP)-II. Agency for Health Research and Quality, Washington, DC

American Academy of Pediatrics & American College of Obstetricians and Gynecologists (1997) *Guidelines for Perinatal Care*. 4 edn. ACOG,

American College of Nurse-Midwives (2004) *Unnecessary Episiotomies: The Nurse-Midwifery Solution*. www.midwife.org/prof/display.cfm?id=87 (accessed on 15 June 2004)

Anderson S (1977) Childbirth as a pathological process: an American perspective. *Am J Maternal Child Nurs* July/ August: 240–4

Anonymous (1968) Episiotomy. *The Lancet* 13 January: 75–6

Anonymous (1976) Episiotomy — the unkindest cut. *AIMS Quarterly Newsletter* March: 7

Anonymous (1993) Mothers who use nurse midwives have fewer C-sections, episiotomies and shorter hospital stays. *J Nurs Administration* **23**: 11–12

Anonymous (1994) Reducing Episiotomy. Editorial. *Accoucher: A Newsletter for Primary Care in Childbirth* 1 April: 3

Argentine Episiotomy Trial Collaborative Group (1993) Routine vs selective episiotomy: a randomised controlled trial. Argentine Episiotomy Trial Collaborative Group. *The Lancet* **342**(8886–8887): 1517–18

Australian Institute of Health and Welfare, and National Perinatal Statistics Unit (2001) *Australia's Mothers and Babies 1999*. AIHW National Perinatal Statistics Unit, 2nd floor, McNevin Dickson Building, Randwick Hospitals Campus, Avoca Street, Randwick, NSW 2031

Australian Institute of Health and Welfare, and National Perinatal Statistics Unit (2003) *Australia's Mothers and Babies 2000*. AIHW National Perinatal Statistics Unit, 2nd floor, McNevin Dickson Building, Randwick Hospitals Campus, Avoca Street, Randwick, NSW 2031

Barros FC, Victora CG, Horta BL (2001) Ethnicity and infant health in Southern Brazil. A birth cohort study. *Int J Epidemiol* **30**(5): 1001–8

Begley CM (2002) Consumer demand for caesarean sections in Brazil. Episiotomy rates may change after evidence based intervention. *Br Med J* **325**(7359): 335

Belizan JM, Carroli G (1998) Routine episiotomy should be abandoned. *Br Med J* **317**(7169): 1389

Board on Global Health and Institute of Medicine (2003) *Improving Birth Outcomes: Meeting the Challenge in the Developing World*. National Academies Press, Washington, DC

Bodner-Adler B, Bodner K, Kaider A, Wagenbichler P, Leodolter S, Husslein P, Mayerhofer K (2001) Risk factors for third-degree perineal tears in vaginal delivery, with an analysis of episiotomy types. *J Reprod Med* **46**(8): 752–6

Bodner-Adler B, Bodner K, Kimberger O, Wagenbichler P, Mayerhofer K (2003) Management of the perineum during forceps delivery. Association of episiotomy with the frequency and severity of perineal trauma in women undergoing forceps delivery. *J Reprod Med* **48**(4): 239–42

Boston Women's Health Collective (1973) *Our Bodies, Ourselves: A Book by and for Women*. Simon and Schuster, New York

Bourget M, Ymayo M (2000) Changes in the delivery room: An alternative way to reduce the C-section rate and episiotomy rate in a Brazilian hospital. *Int J Gynaecol Obstet* **70**(S2): B86

Brink PJ (1982) Traditional birth attendants among the Annang of Nigeria : Current practices and proposed programs. *Soc Sci Med* **16**(21): 1883–92

Brody H, Thompson J (1981) The Maximin Strategy in Modern Obstetrics. *J Fam Pract* **12**(6): 977–86

Bruce E (2001) Saying no to episiotomy: Getting through labour in one piece. *Mothering* Jan-Feb. http://www.findarticles.com/p/articles/mi_m0838/is_2001_Jan-Feb/ai_76587453 (accessed 27 October 2004)

Carroli G, Belizan J (2004) *Episiotomy for vaginal birth*. The Cochrane Library 2004 Issue 4. John Wiley & Sons Ltd, Chichester, UK

Carvalho I, Chacham AS, Viana P (1998) Traditional birth attendants and their practices in the State of Pernambuco rural area, Brazil, 1996. *Int J Gynaecol Obstet* **63**(suppl 1): S53–S60

Chalmers B (1995) Psychosomatic obstetrics in the countries of Central and Eastern Europe. *J Psychosomatic Obstet Gynecol* **16**: 59–63

Chalmers B, Muggah H, Samarskaya MF, Tkatchenko E (1998) Women's experiences of birth in St Petersburg, Russian Federation, following a maternal and child health intervention program. *Birth* **25**(2): 107

Chalmers I (1975) *Evaluation of different apporaches to obstetric care*. Paper presented at Warwick University, 10 October 1975

CLAP (2004) Best Practices for Labor and Perinatal Care: A Special Award Program to Maternities that Provide High Quality Services for Mothers and Children. www.paho.org/English/CLAP/invpro14.htm. CLAP, PAHO, WHO (accessed 15 June 2004)

Coats PM, Chan KK, Wilkins M, Beard RJ (1980) A comparison between midline and mediolateral episiotomies. *Br J Obstet Gynaecol* **87**(5): 408–12

Cravchik S, Munoz DM, Bortman M (1998) Indications for episiotomy at public maternity clinics in Nequen, Argentina. *Rev Panam Salud Publica* **4**(1): 26–31

Cuidiu (1999) *Preparing Together for Birth and Beyond: A Consumer Guide to the Maternity Services in Ireland*. Irish Childbirth Trust, Dublin

Cunningham F, Gant N, Leveno K, Gilstrap L, Hauth J, Wenstrom K (2001) *Williams Obstetrics*. 21 edn. McGraw-Hill, New York

Dannecker C, Hillemanns P, Strauss A, Hasbargen U, Hepp H, Anthuber C (2004) Episiotomy and perineal tears presumed to be imminent: randomized controlled trial. *Acta Obstet Gynecol Scand* 83(4): 364–8

David M, von Schwarzenfeld H, Dimer JAS, Kentenich H (1999) Perinatal outcome in hospital and birth center obstetric care. *Int J Gynecol Obstet* **65**(2): 149–56

David M (1993) Who invented the episiotomy? On the history of the episiotomy. *Zentralbl Gynakol* **115**(4): 188–93

Davis F (1976) Who's having the baby — you or the doctor? *Women's Day* 10 March: 146–52

Davis-Floyd RE (1990) The role of obstetrical rituals in the resolution of cultural anomaly. *Soc Sci Med* **31**(2): 175–89

Declerq, Eugene R, Sakala, Carol, Corry, Maureen P (2002) *Listening to Mothers: Report of the First National US Survey of Women's Childbearing Experiences.* Maternity Center Association, Harris Interactive

DeLee JB (1920) The prophylactic forceps operation. Read before the 45th Annual Meeting of the American Gynecological Society, 24–26 May 1920. *Am J Obstet Gynecol* **1**: 24–44

Diani F, Zanconato G, Foschi F, Turinetto A, Franchi M (2003) Management of the pregnant immigrant woman in the decade 1992–2001. *J Obstet Gynaecol* **23**(6): 615–17

Dimitrov A, Nalbanski B, Nikolov A, Stamenov G, Dimitrov I, Lazarova L, Gamishev G (1997) An analysis of the indications for episiotomy in current obstetrical practice. *Akush Ginekol (Sofiia)* **36**(1): 1–3

Diniz SG, Chacham AS (2004) 'The Cut Above' and 'the Cut Below': The abuse of Caesareans and episiotomy in Sao Paulo, Brazil. *Reproductive Health Matters* **12**(23): 100–10

Eason E, Feldman P (2000) Much ado about a little cut: is episiotomy worthwhile? *Obstet Gynecol* **95**(4): 616–18

Eason E, Labrecque M, Marcoux S, Mondor M (2002) Anal incontinence after childbirth. *CMAJ* **166**(3): 326–30

Eberhard J, Geissbuehler V (2000) Influence of alternative birth methods on traditional birth management. *Fetal Diagnosis and Therapy* **15**: 283–90

Eltorkey M, Al Nuaim M, Kurdi A, Sabagh T, Clarke F (1994) Episiotomy, elective or selective: a report of a random allocation trial. *J Obstet Gynaecol* **14**: 317–20

England and Government Statistical Service (2004) *NHS Maternity Statistics, England: 2002–03*

Enkin M, Keirs M, Chalmers I (1989) *A Guide to Effective Care in Pregnancy and Childbirth.* Oxford University Press, New York

Enkin M, Kerice M, Neilson J, Duley L, Hodnett E, Hofmeyr J (2004) The second stage of labor. In: *A Guide to Effective Care in Pregnancy and Childbirth.* 3rd edn. Oxford University Press, Oxford

Flint C, Poulengeris P, Grant A (1989) The 'Know Your Midwife' scheme — a randomised trial of continuity of care by a team of midwives. *Midwifery* **5**(1): 11–16

Fraser C (1983) Selected perinatal procedures. Scientific basis for the use of psychosocial effects. A literature review. *Acta Obstetricia et Gynecologica Scandinavica* **117**: 5–39

Froshaug J (1974) The unkindest cut of all? *Nova* September: 84–5

Gerrits D, Brand R, Bennebroek Gravenhorst J (1994) The use of episiotomy in relation to the professional education of the delivery attendant. *Eur J Obstet Gynecol Reproductive Biology* **56**: 103–06

Goldberg J, Holtz D, Hyslop T, Tolosa JE (2002) Has the use of routine episiotomy decreased? Examination of episiotomy rates from 1983 to 2000. *Obstet Gynecol* **99**(3): 395–400

Graham ID (1996) I believe therefore I practise. *The Lancet* **347**(8993): 4–5

Graham ID, Fowler-Graham D (1997a) Episiotomy counts: trends and prevalence in Canada, 1981/1982 to 1993/1994. *Birth* **24**(3): 141–7

Graham ID (1997b) *Episiotomy: Challenging Obstetric Interventions*. Blackwell Science, Oxford

Graham ID (1998) Processes of change in obstetrics: a cross-national case-study of episiotomy. *Health* **2**(4): 403–33

Graham SB, Catanzarite V, Bernstein J, Varela-Gittings F (1990) A comparison of attitudes and practices of episiotomy among obstetrical practitioners in New Mexico. *Soc Sci Med* **31**(2): 191–201

Griffin N (1995) Avoiding an episiotomy. *Mothering Magazine* **75**: 56

Haire D (1972) *The Cultural Warping of Childbirth*. International Childbirth Education Assocation, Minneapolis, Minnesota

Harrison R, Brennan M, North P, Reed J, Wickham E (1984) Is routine episiotomy necessary? *Br Med J* **288**: 1971–75

Harvey S, Jarrell J, Brant R, Stainton C, Rach D (1996) A randomized, controlled trial of nurse-midwifery care. *Birth* **23**(3): 128–35

Health Canada (2000) *Family-Centred Maternity and Newborn Care: National Guidelines*. Minister of Public Works and Government Services, Ottawa

Health Canada (2003) *Canadian Perinatal Health Report 2003*. Minister of Public Works and Government Services Canada

Helwig JT, Thorp JM Jr, Bowes WA Jr (1993) Does midline episiotomy increase the risk of third- and fourth-degree lacerations in operative vaginal deliveries? *Obstet Gynecol* **82**(2): 276–9

Henriksen TB, Bek KM, Hedegaard M, Secher NJ (1992) Episiotomy and perineal lesions in spontaneous vaginal deliveries. *Br J Obstet Gynaecol* **99**(12): 950–4

Henriksen TB, Bek KM, Hedegaard M, Secher NJ (1994) Methods and consequences of changes in use of episiotomy. *Br Med J* **309**: 1255–58

Heres MHB, Pel M, Elferink-Stinkens PM, Van Hemel OJS, Treffers PE (1995) The Dutch obstetric intervention study — variations in practice patterns. *Int J Gynecol Obstet* **50**(2): 145–50

Hirsch HA (1997) Episiotomy and its complications. *Z Geburtshilfe Neonatol* **201**(suppl 1): 55–62

Hirst B (1902) *A Text-book of Obstetrics*. 3rd edn. WB Saunders and Company, Philadelphia

Hodnett ED (1999) Continuity of Caregivers for Care During Pregnancy and Childbirth. The Cochrane Library 2004 Issue 4. John Wiley & Sons Ltd, Chichester, UK

House M (1981) Episiotomy — indications, techniques and results. *Midwife, Health Visitor, and Community Nurse* **17**: 6–9

House M, Cario G, Jones M (1986) Episiotomy and the perineum: a random controlled trial. *J Obstet Gynaecol* **7**: 107–10

Howard D, Davies PS, DeLancey JO, Small Y (2000) Differences in perineal lacerations in black and white primiparas. *Obstet Gynecol* **96**(4): 622–4

Howden NLS, Weber AM, Meyn LA (2004) Episiotomy Use Among Residents and Faculty Compared With Private Practitioners. *Obstet Gynecol* **103**(1): 114–18

Hueston WJ (1996) Factors associated with the use of episiotomy during vaginal delivery. *Obstet Gynecol* **87**(6): 1001–1005

Hundley V, Cruickshank F, Lang G, Glazener C, Milne J, Turner M *et al* (1994) Midwife managed delivery unit: a randomised controlled comparison iwth consultant led care. *Br Med J* **309**: 1400–04

Jander C, Lyrenas S (2001) Third and fourth degree perineal tears. Predictor factors in a referral hospital. *Acta Obstet Gynecol Scand* **80**(3): 229–34

Kaczorowski J, Levitt C, Hanvey L, Avard D, Chance G (1998) A national survey of use of obstetric procedures and technologies in Canadian hospitals: routine or based on existing evidence? *Birth* **25**(1): 11–18

Kaufman K, MacDonald H (1988) A retrospective evaluation of a model of midwifery care. *Birth* **15**: 95–9

Kitzinger S (1972) *Episiotomy: Physical and Emotional Aspects*. National Childbirth Trust, London

Kitzinger S (1979) *Episiotomy. Controversy*. Midwife, Health Visitor, and Community Nurse **15**(6): 233–4

Kitzinger S (1981) *Episiotomy: Physical and Emotional Aspects*. 2nd edn. National Childbirth Trust, London

Kitzinger S (1999) Sheila Kitzinger's letter from Europe: obstetric metaphors and marketing. *Birth* **26**(1): 55–7

Kitzinger S, Walters R (1981) *Some Women's Experiences of Episiotomy*. National Childbirth Trust, London

Klein MC, Gauthier RJ, Robbins JM, Kaczorowski J, Jorgensen SH, Franco ED *et al* (1994) Relationship of episiotomy to perineal trauma and morbidity, sexual dysfunction, and pelvic floor relaxation. *Am J Obstet Gynecol* **171**(3): 591–8

Klein MC, Kaczorowski J, Robbins JM, Gauthier RJ, Jorgensen SH, Joshi AK (1995) Physicians' beliefs and behaviour during a randomized controlled trial of episiotomy: consequences for women in their care. *CMAJ* **153**(6): 769–79

Klein M, Gauthier R, Jorgensen SH, Robbins JM, Kaczorowski J (1992) Does episiotomy prevent perineal trauma and pelvic floor relaxation? *Online J Curr Clinical Trials* **10**: 1 July

Kolbl H (2001) Pregnancy, childbirth and the pelvic floor. *Zentralbl Gynakol* **123**(12): 666–71

Kozak LJ, Dawson Weeks J (2002) US Trends in Obstetric Procedures, 1990–2000. *Birth* **29**: 157–61

Kozak LJ, Hall MJ, Owings MF (2002) National Hospital Discharge Survey: 2000 annual summary with detailed diagnosis and procedure data

Labrecque M, Baillargeon L, Dallaire M, Tremblay A, Pinault JJ, Gingras S (1997) Association between median episiotomy and severe perineal lacerations in primiparous women. *CMAJ*, **156**(6): 797–802

Levett D (1974) Episiotomy — an overused procedure? Open Forum. *Nurs Mirror* 17 October: 89

Lorenz N, Nougtara A, Garner P (1998) Episiotomy in Burkina Faso. *Trop Doct* **28**(2): 83–5

Low LK, Seng JS, Murtland TL, Oakley D (2000) Clinician-specific episiotomy rates: impact on perineal outcomes. *J Midwifery Womens Health* **45**(2): 87–93

Maier KM (2000) *The Pregnancy Planning Guide: An Evidence-Based Guide to Pregnancy*. Children's and Women's Health Centre of British Columbia, Vancouver

Manzer J (2002) No science behind use of episiotomy. *Medical Post* **38**(10): 3–12

Marcus A (2004) Episiotomy Rates Dropping in US. *Health Day* 7 May

Mehl L (1978) Scientific research on childbirth alternatives: what can it tell us about 20th century hospital practice. In: Stewart L, Stewart D, eds. *21st Century Obstetrics Now!* volume 1. NAPSAC, Marble Hill, Missouri: 171–208

MNH (2004) *Guatemala's Clinical Skills Training Fosters New Practices and Attitudes.* www.mnh.jhpiego.org/news/guatcst.asp (accessed 15 June 2004)

Morris N (1981) A very common operation. Editorial. *Midwife, Health Visitor, and Community Nurse* **901**: 243

Newman M, Lidsay M, Graves W (2001) The effect of epidural analgesia on rates of episiotomy use and episiotomy extension in an inner-city hospital. *J Materal-Fetal Health* **10**(2): 97–101

NSW Health Department (1997) NSW Mothers and Babies Report 1997. http://www.mhcs.health.nsw.gov.au/pubs/m/pdf/mdcrep97.pdf (accessed 15 June 2004)

Page L, McCourt C, Beake S, Vail A, Hewiston J (1999) Clinical interventions and outcomes of one-to-one midwifery practice. *J Public Health Med* **21**(3): 243–8

Panter G (1980) Episiotomy: the question of informed consent. *Parents* May: 86–8

Pomeroy RH (1918) Shall we cut and reconstruct the perineum for every primipara? Paper read before the American Gynecological Society, 16–18 May 1918. *Am J Obstet Dis Women and Children* **78**: 211–20

Qian X, Smith H, Zhou L, Liang J, Garner P (2001) Evidence-based obstetrics in four hospitals in China: An observational study to explore clinical practice, women's preferences and provider's views. *BMC Pregnancy Childbirth* **1**(1): 1

Rageth JC, Buerklen A, Hirsch HA (1989) [Late complications of episiotomy.] *Z Geburtshilfe Perinatol* 193(5): 233–7

Rana TG, Rajopadhyaya R, Bajracharya B, Karmacharya M, Osrin D (2003) Comparison of midwifery-led and consultant-led maternity care for low risk deliveries in Nepal. *Health Policy Plan* **18**(3): 330–7

Ratner H (1978) History of the dehumanization of American obstetrical practice. In: Stewart L, Stewart D, eds. *21st Century Obstetrics Now!* NAPSAC, Marble Hill, Missouri: 115–46

Reynolds JL (1995) Reducing the frequency of episiotomies through a continuous quality improvement program. *CMAJ* **153**(3): 275–82

Richards T (2004) Poor countries lack relevant health information. *Br Med J* **328**: 310

Riskin-Mashiah S, O'Brian SE, Wilkins IA (2002) Risk factors for severe perineal tear: can we do better? *Am J Perinatol* **19**(5): 225–34

Robinson JN, Norwitz ER, Cohen AP, Lieberman E (2000) Predictors of episiotomy use at first spontaneous vaginal delivery. *Obstet Gynecol* 96: 214–8

Robinson JN, Norwitz ER, Cohen AP, Lieberman E (2001) Risk factors for episiotomy. *ACOG Clinical Review* **6**(1): 3–4

Robinson JN, Norwitz ER, Cohen AP, Lieberman E (2000) Predictors of episiotomy use at first spontaneous vaginal delivery. *Obstet Gynecol* **96**(2): 214–18

Rockner G, Fianu-Jonasson A (1999) Changed pattern in the use of episiotomy in Sweden. *Br J Obstet Gynaecol* **106**(2): 95–101

Rockner G, Olund A (1991) The use of episiotomy in primiparas in Sweden. A descriptive study with particular focus on two hospitals. *Acta Obstet Gynecol Scand* **70**(4–5): 325–30

Rowley MJ, Hensley MJ, Brinsmead MW, Wlodarczyk JH (1995) Continuity of care by a midwife team versus routine care during pregnancy and birth: a randomised trial. *Med J Aust* **163**(6): 289–93

Royal College of Obstetricians and Gynaecologists (2000) *Methods and Materials used in Perineal Repair.* www.rcog.org.uk/guidelines.asp?PageID=106%GuidelineID=15 (accessed 15 June 2004)

Royal College of Obstetricians and Gynaecologists (2002) *Maternal Morbidity and Mortality — Study Group Recommendations*. www.rcog.org.uk/mainpages.asp?PageID=908 (accessed 15 June 2004)

Russell J (1982) Episiotomy. Editorial. *Br Med J* **284**: 220

Sartore A, De Seta F, Maso G, Pregazzi R, Grimaldi E, Guaschino S (2004) The effects of mediolateral episiotomy on pelvic floor function after vaginal delivery. *Obstet Gynecol* **103**(4): 669–73

Schlomer G, Gross M, Meyer G (2003) [Effectiveness of liberal vs. conservative episiotomy in vaginal delivery with reference to preventing urinary and fecal incontinence: a systematic review]. *Wien Med Wochenschr* **153**(11–12): 269–75

Shiono P, Klebanoff MA, Carey JC (1990) Midline episiotomies: more harm than good? *Obstet Gynecol* **75**(5): 765–70

Shorten A, Shorten B (2000) Women's choice? The impact of private health insurance on episiotomy rates in Australian hospitals. *Midwifery* **16**(3): 204–12

Shute W (1959) Episiotomy: A physiologic appraisal and new painless technic. *Obstet Gynecol* **14**(4): 467–72

Signorello LB, Harlow BL, Chekos AK, Repke JT (2000) Midline episiotomy and anal incontinence: retrospective cohort study. *Br Med J* **320**(7227): 86–90

Simpson K, Knox G (1999) Strategies for developing an evidence-based approach to perinatal care. *MCN* **24**(3): 122–32

Sleep J (1987) Perineal management — a midwifery skill under threat. *Midwife, Health Visitor, and Community Nurse* **23**(20): 455–8

Sleep J, Grant A, Garcia J, Elbourne D, Spencer J, Chalmers I (1984) West Berkshire perineal management trial. *Br Med J* **289**: 587–90

Sleep J, Roberts J, Chalmers I (1989) Care during the second stage of labour. In: Chalmers I, Enkins M, Keirse M, eds. *Effective Care in Pregnancy and Childbirth*. Oxford University Press, Oxford: 1136–44

Smith H, Brown H, Hofmeyr J, Garner P, Rees H, Dickson-Tetteh K (2001) *Better Birth Initiative: South Africa pilot study report*. Cochrane Colloquium meeting abstract book 1: b057, Lyon, France

Smith H, Mahomed K, Hofmeyr J, Nikodem C, Garner P (1999) *Getting research into practice: women-centred obstetric care*. 7th Annual Cochrane Colloquium, Rome

Smith M, Ruffin M, Green L (1993) The rational management of labour. *Am Fam Phys* **47**: 1471–81

Society of Obstetricians and Gynaecologists of Canada (1998) *Clinical Practice Guidelines: Healthy Beginnings for Care During Pregnancy and Childbirth*. SOGC, Ottawa

Stotland NL (2004) Women's bodies, doctors' dynamics. *J Am Acad Psychoanal Dyn Psychiatry* **32**(1): 181–91

Stratton J, Gordon H, Logue M (1995) Conclusions and validity of data cannot be judged. *Br Med J* **310**: 668

Taylor E (1982) Editorial Note. *Obstetr Gynecol Surv* **37**(10): 614

Thacker SB (2000) Midline versus mediolateral episiotomy. *Br Med J* **320**(7250): 1615–16

Thacker SB, Banta HD (1983) Benefits and risks of episiotomy: an interpretative review of the English language literature, 1860–1980. *Obstet Gynecol Surv* **38**(6): 322–38

Tincello DG, Williams A, Fowler GE, Adams EJ, Richmond DH, Alfirevic Z (2003) Differences in episiotomy technique between midwives and doctors. *Br J Obstet Gynaecol* **110**(12): 1041–44

Turnbull D, Holmes A, Shields N, Cheyne H, Twaddle S, Gilmour WH *et al* (1996) Randomised, controlled trial of efficacy of midwife-managed care. *Lancet* **348**(9022): 213–18

US National Library of Medicine (2004) *Improving perinatal care in Latin America.* http://www.clinicaltrials.gov/show/NCT00070720 (accessed 6 April 2004)

Wagner M (1994) *Pursuing the birth machine. The search for appropriate technology.* ACE Graphics, Camperdown, New South Wales

Weber AM, Meyn L (2002) Episiotomy use in the United States, 1979-1997. *Obstet Gynecol* **100**(6): 1177–82

Weeks JD, Kozak LJ (2001) Trends in the use of episiotomy in the United States: 1980–1998. *Birth* **28**(3): 152–60

Werner C, Schuler W, Meskendahl I (1991) Midline episiotomy versus medio-lateral episiotomy. A randomized prospective study. Proceedings of 13th World Congress of Gynaecology and Obstetrics (FIGO), Singapore, Book 1:33

World Health Organization (1996) *Care during second stage of labour. Care in normal birth.* www.who.int/reproductive-health/publications [4] (accessed 15 June 2004)

World Health Organization Procedures (2000) *Managing Complications in Pregnancy and Childbirth: A guide for midwives and doctors.* www.who.int/reproductive-health/impac/procedures/episiotomy_P71_P75.html [3] (accessed 15 June 2004)

WHO and PAHO (1985) Appropriate Technology for Birth. *Lancet* **326**(8452): 436–7

Wilkerson V (1984) The use of episiotomy in normal delivery. *Midwives Chronicle and Nursing Notes*, April: 106–10

Williams FL, du VF, Mires GJ, Ogston SA (1998) Episiotomy and perineal tears in low-risk UK primigravidae. *J Public Health Med* **20**(4): 422–7

Willmot J (1979) No need to flaw the pelvic floor. Viewpoint. *Nursing Mirror* 29 March: 31

Woolley RJ (1995a) Benefits and risks of episiotomy: a review of the English-language literature since 1980. Part I. *Obstet Gynecol Surv* **50**(11): 806–20

Woolley RJ (1995b) Benefits and risks of episiotomy: a review of the English-language literature since 1980. Part II. *Obstet Gynecol Surv* **50**(11): 821–35

Yeh PS (2002) Childbirth in Taiwan is certainly overmedicalized. *Br Med J* **325**: 103

Yunker B (1975) Delivery procedures that endanger a baby's life. Are doctors interfering too much with the natural process of giving birth? Many women — and some leading obstetricians — feel that they are. *Good Housekeeping* **181**[August]: 56–61

Zander L (1982) Episiotomy: has familiarity bred contempt? Editorial. *J Roy Coll Gen Pract* **32**(July): 400–1

Zondervan KT, Buitendijk SE, Anthony S, van Rijssel EJ, Verkerk PH (1995) [Frequency and determinants of episiotomy in second-line obstetrics in The Netherlands]. *Ned Tijdschr Geneeskd* **139**(9): 449–52

## References to *Table 5.1*

1.  Health Canada (2003) *Canadian Perinatal Health Report 2003.* Minister of Public Works and Government Services Canada. http://www.hc-sc.gc.ca/pphb-dgspsp/rhs-ssg/index.html (accessed 15 June 2004)

2. Kozak LJ, Hall MJ, Owings MF (2002) National Hospital Discharge Survey: 2000 annual summary with detailed diagnosis and procedure data. *Vital Health Stat* **13**(153): 1–194

3. Belizan JM, Carroli G (1998) Routine episiotomy should be abandoned. *Br Med J* **317**: 1389

4. Althabe F, Belizan JM, Bergel E (2002) Episiotomy rates in primiparous women in Latin America: hospital based descriptive study. *Br Med J* **324**: 945–6

5. MNH (2004) *Guatemala's Clinical Skills Training Fosters New Practices and Attitudes.* www.mnh.jhpiego.org/news/guatcst.asp (accessed 15 June 2004)

6. Alran S, Sibony O, Oury JF, Luton D, Blot P (2002) Differences in management and results in term-delivery in nine European referral hospitals: descriptive study. *Eur J Obstet Gynecol Reprod Biol* **103**: 4–13

7. Wildman K, Blondel B, Nijhuis J, Defoort P, Bakoula C (2003) European indicators of health care during pregnancy, delivery and the postpartum period. *Eur J Obstet Gynecol Reprod Biol* **111**(suppl 1): S53–S65

8. Finland and National Research and Development Centre for Welfare and Health (2002) Parturients, births and newborn infants 2002.
http://www.stakes.info/2/1/2,1,1.asp (accessed 15 June 2004)

9. England and Government Statistical Service (2004) NHS Maternity Statistics, England: 2002–03.

10. Pel M, Heres MH, Hart AA, van d, V, Treffers PE (1995) Provider-associated factors in obstetric interventions. *Eur J Obstet Gynecol Reprod Biol* **61**: 129–34

11. Schwappach DL, Blaudszun A, Conen D, Eichler K, Hochreutener MA, Koeck CM (2004) Women's experiences with low-risk singleton in-hospital delivery in Switzerland. *Swiss Med Wkly* **134**: 103–9

12. France. National Perinatal Report. 2004.
http://www.sante.gouv.fr/htm/dossiers/perinat/5_metropole.htm

13. Karacam Z, Eroglu K (2003) Effects of episiotomy on bonding and mothers' health. *J Adv Nurs* **43**: 384–94

14. Garcia EM, Merino MJR, San Martin MLB (1998) Episiotomy in the Hospital General Universitario in Alicante, Spain. Description and evaluation [Spanish]. *Enfermeria Clinica* **8**(1): 1-6

15. Dimitrov A, Nalbanski B, Nikolov A, Stamenov G, Dimitrov I, Lazarova L *et al* (1997) [An analysis of the indications for episiotomy in current obstetrical practice]. *Akush Ginekol* (Sofiia) **36**: 1-3

16. Dimitrov A, Nikolov A, Nalbanski B, Stamenov G, Dimitrov I, Lazarova L et al (1997) [The results of the limited use of episiotomy in managing the second stage of labor]. *Akush Ginekol* (Sofiia.) **36**: 3–4

17. Chalmers B, Muggah H, Samarskaya MF, Tkatchenko E (1998) Women's Experiences of Birth in St. Petersburg, Russian Federation, Following a Maternal and Child Health Intervention Program. *Birth* **25**: 107

18. Rana TG, Rajopadhyaya R, Bajracharya B, Karmacharya M, Osrin D (2003) Comparison of midwifery-led and consultant-led maternity care for low risk deliveries in Nepal. *Health Policy Plan* **18**: 330–7

19. Qian X, Smith H, Zhou L, Liang J, Garner P (2001) Evidence-based obstetrics in four hospitals in China: An observational study to explore clinical practice, women's preferences and provider's views. *BMC Pregnancy Childbirth* **1**: 1

20. Yeh PS (2002) Childbirth in Taiwan is certainly overmedicalized. *Br Med J* **325**: 103
21. Jakobi P (2001) Episiotomy: An unkind and unnecessary cut. http://www.perinatology2001.com (accessed 15 June 2004)
22. New Zealand Ministry of Health and New Zealand Health Information Service (2003) *Report on Maternity 2000 and 2001*. New Zealand Health Information Service
23. Shorten A, Shorten B (2000) Women's choice? The impact of private health insurance on episiotomy rates in Australian hospitals. *Midwifery* **16**: 204–12
24. Australian Institute of Health and Welfare and National Perinatal Statistics Unit (2003) *Australia's Mothers and Babies 2000*. AIHW National Perinatal Statistics Unit, 2nd floor, McNevin Dickson Building, Randwick Hospitals Campus, Avoca Street, Randwick, NSW 2031, Australia, National Perinatal Statistics Unit.
25. Lorenz N, Nougtara A, Garner P (1998) Episiotomy in Burkina Faso. *Trop Doct* **28**: 83–5
26. Oyo-Ita A, Ekott M, Chiazor H, Meremikwu M (2001) *Better Birth Initiative — Calabar project*. Cochrane Colloquium meeting abstract book 1: b064, Lyon, France
27. Pfau R (2001) Audit on Obstetrical Care in the Maternity Ward of Bamalete Lutheran Hospital, Ramotswa, Botswana http://www.perinatalpriorities.co.za/dbfiles/Priorities20%20-%202001.doc (accessed 15 June 2004)
28. van den Bergh JE, Sueters M, Segaar M, van Roosmalen J (2003) Determinants of episiotomy in rural Zimbabwe. *Acta Obstet Gynecol Scand* **82**: 966–8
29. Pattinson R, Howarrth G, Mdluli W, Macdonald A, Makin J, Funk M (2003) Aggressive or expectant management of labour: a randomized clinical trial. *Br J Obstet Gynaecol* **110**: 457–61

## 6

# Perineal tear assessment and the development of the Peri-Rule™

*Susan Tohill and Alison Metcalfe*

## Introduction

Some of the previous chapters have focused on the problems encountered by women once they have sustained perineal trauma and the effect it can have on their quality of life for weeks, months or even years. Following some pilot work taking place across several maternity units in Birmingham, England, midwives and researchers (who formed the Birmingham Perineal Research Evaluation Group), noted the lack of an objective assessment and measurement of perineal trauma.

The majority of individual midwives in the UK follow the guidelines of the Royal College of Midwives (RCM) and Royal College of Obstetricians and Gynaecologists (RCOG) on the classification of perineal tears. This classification ranges from first to fourth degree (as described in *Chapter 4*). However, there was no system of classifying the actual size of tear, which could be highly variable, ranging from a few millimetres to several centimetres in size. Unless a maternity unit has a local policy of suturing all second- degree tears, most midwives rely on their own and colleagues professional experience in deciding at which point the perineal tear is too large to leave unsutured.

Up until the early 1990s, all second-degree tears were sutured by an obstetrician and it was a general policy of most maternity units to repair perineal tears. Following the publication of small, retrospective studies (Head, 1993; Clement and Reed, 1999) some midwives began to question the need to suture second-degree tears particularly 'smaller' ones. However, this raises the question: what is a 'small', 'medium' or 'large' second-degree perineal tear?

The highly subjective nature of describing second-degree perineal trauma and the current trend in practice to leave some second-degree tears unsutured, means that a method of measuring the tears is required. Otherwise, how do you assess the outcomes of the care for women you carry out, either suturing or non-suturing? How do you teach student midwives about assessment of perineal trauma and provide objective guidelines for distinguishing between different sizes of tear? Finally, how can you undertake research into comparing the effectiveness of suturing or non-suturing if you cannot be certain that you are comparing second-degree perineal tears of a similar size? An objective method of measuring second-degree tears is required to assist audit, education and research in midwifery practice.

One of the main reasons that a major randomised controlled trial to compare suturing versus non-suturing of second-degree tears has not taken place is because there has never been a reliable method of measuring and assessing trauma to the perineum. Perineal tears are generally classified by the anatomical tissues involved. A second-degree tear is classified as involving perineal muscle, vaginal wall and skin (RCOG Guideline 23, 2004). There are no indications on the actual size of tear, which can vary greatly in length and depth. Comparisons between sutured tears and non-sutured tears without assessment of size would be unreliable and it may be that one size of tear is better left unsutured than another. Plus, any cohort studies that monitor the outcomes without randomising 'treatment' options, are also prone to bias because larger tears are more likely to be sutured than smaller tears (Metcalfe *et al*, 2002). If size comparisons cannot be made between sutured and unsutured perineal tears, this would obviously be a major flaw in any research project.

## Previous perineal trauma assessment tools

There have been a number of tools developed for the assessment of perineal trauma. The development of a reliable tool for measuring tears, however, has been difficult. These tools vary in their objective; some have the principal aim of measuring perineal trauma whilst most assessments have focused on postpartum healing of the perineum, following a tear or episiotomy.

The first systematic attempt to evaluate postpartum healing of the perineum was the REEDA tool devised by Davidson (1970) with revisions by Carey (1971) and Bolles (1972) (cited in Davidson, 1974). The tool examined five components of the healing process, the amount of redness (R), Edema (E), Ecchymosis of the perineal area (E), level of discharge from wound (D) and approximation of the skin edges at the site of episiotomy (A).

In each category there is a scale of four points from 0–3, with 0 indicating nil trauma and 3 indicating the most trauma. The category scores are added together to produce an overall score which can range from 0–15.

The REEDA tool involved cutting disposable paper tapes into 4cm lengths, which had 0.25cm divisions marked out. Whilst the woman is in a lateral Sims position, tape is placed perpendicular to the line of incision so that its mid portion centimetre marking is aligned with the incision. Each side of the episiotomy is measured precisely in relation to their proximity to the incision.

Since its development, the REEDA tool has only been used to a limited extent. The main reasons appear to be due to intrusiveness and a complicated system of using paper tape that is easily soiled and difficult to align especially when measuring bruising (Steen and Cooper, 1997). The use of the REEDA tool in the community setting was particularly limited because of the positioning of women, relatively poor lighting and usually no assistance was available.

Hill (1990) devised the perineal assessment tool (PAT) to test whether the REEDA tool would be clinically useful to assess trauma. The perineal assessment tool assessed redness, swelling, bruising, drainage and suture line with a categorical scoring system of non present, small, moderate and severe. Following testing, which involved assessing the level of consistency in scores being obtained between two independent assessors (raters), the tool was not reliable. The categorical scoring system was too subjective resulting in low reliability and therefore use in clinical practice was not advised (Hill, 1990).

Another tool developed by Steen and Cooper (1997) used photographs to guide assessment. The principal aim was to identify a visual non-intrusive method for measuring perineal oedema and bruising in order to investigate the effectiveness of a new maternity gel pad. Due to difficulties with the photographs, a categorical scoring scale, modified from the REEDA tool, was used to assess bruising and oedema. Instead of using a tape to measure the trauma, a visual non-touch finger measurement was adopted, using the basis that the width of a little finger represented 1cm. The tool has not been extensively investigated for its reliability in assessing bruising and oedema and preliminary work showed that there was some variation in reliability, particularly between experienced and newly qualified midwives.

Photographs were also used by Gomme *et al* (2001) who developed a tool initially based on photographic depictions of different types and sizes of trauma and asking midwives to rate the severity. Briefly the study of Gomme *et al* (2001) was carried out in three phases.

After gaining individual women's consent, phase 1 involved taking photographs depicting different types of perineal tears. However, Gomme *et al* (2001) explain that the lack of three-dimensional images from the photograph meant the depth of perineal trauma could not be assessed. For phase 2, focus group discussions with hospital and community midwives were held to ask these professionals to articulate what criteria, with reference to the photographs, they used to assess perineal trauma and decide whether a tear required suturing. This information was used to develop an assessment tool for the final phase.

The third phase involved the testing of the tool by two midwife raters examining fifty-two women that had sustained perineal trauma. In carrying out tests for statistical reliability the only measurement that had a degree of reliability was the assessment of the distance of the tear from the anus. (The raters had to assess whether the tear was more than or less than 1cm of reaching the anal margin.) This measurement had a kappa score of $\kappa = 0.611$ showing good agreement, whereas the other measurements achieved no agreement (Ullman *et al*, 2004).

Dean *et al* (verbal communication, 2000) reported on the development of a method which involved using artery forceps as a type of sterile callipers to measure the perineal tears. The midwife extends the callipers across the length of the wound and then measures the distance between the calliper points against a tape measure. From the preliminary data communicated, there were fairly good levels of agreement between two midwife raters. However, the numbers of participants involved were insufficient to provide statistically significant evidence of the reliability of the method.


## Development of the Peri-Rule™

Whilst undertaking an epidemiological study to compare the effectiveness of suturing versus non-suturing of second-degree tears, to determine the primary and secondary outcome measures to be used in a randomised trial, 'The Birmingham Perineal Research Evaluation Group' developed the Peri-Rule™ as a means to measure second-degree perineal tears.

The development of the Peri-Rule™ provides the first pragmatic tool for the measurement and assessment of perineal tears. The tool consists of a measuring device and assessment pro forma. The measuring device is made of medical grade, soft plastic with a millimetre scale imprinted on one side (*Figure 6.1*). The single use device is 105mm long, 10mm wide and 4mm in depth and can be cleaned and autoclaved at

130°C for three minutes without any shrinkage or distortion to the scale. The scale is moulded into the plastic, so the device feels smooth to the touch and will not cause any discomfort for the woman or further damage to the wound.

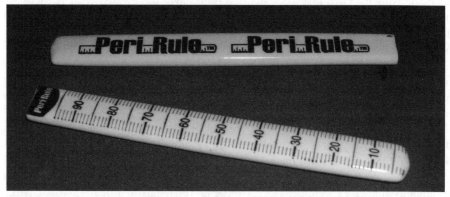

**Figure 6.1: Peri-Rule™. Photograph reproduced by kind permissionof Birmingham Health Science Devices Limited**

The assessment pro forma (*Figure 6.2*) is a set of questions on assessing perineal tears with guidance on the measurements to be taken with the measuring device. It was developed in consultation with practising midwives from each of the five maternity units that formed part of the Birmingham Perineal Research Evaluation Group. The pro forma was devised so that midwives could easily follow a set of simple questions asking midwives about the tear whilst they are realigning the wound edges and assessing the wound. The pro forma is designed to guide the midwife through each stage of assessment of the perineal tear. Each section highlights points that midwives felt were important in evaluating the trauma and may affect their decision-making about advice they would give to the woman. The following sections are included:

1. Overview of guidelines on first-, second-, third- and fourth-degree tears from RCOG and RCM Clinical Green Top Guidelines. This provides the midwife a quick reference point for the guidelines.
2. The positioning of the woman during examination was considered very important; as lithotomy position would usually provide the best view of the tear but there may be instances where this cannot be used.
3. A record of the perineum tissues affected is requested along with a classification of the degree rating, ie. first, second, third or fourth degree.
4. Classification of the second-degree tear based on midwives assessment, ie. is the tear small, medium or large?
5. Record of whether the tear is bleeding.
6. Record of whether the tear is to be sutured along with a record of decision-making by the woman involved and the midwife.
7. Three diagrams that request the midwife to measure the tear in a specific order followed by a section to describe other tears and their complexity.
8. A section for detailing other tears or more complex trauma.

The three diagrams on the pro forma are provided to indicate clearly the measurements required and midwives are advised to measure in a specific order to reduce the risk of infection through the transmission of bacteria into the perineal body. The measurements are requested in the following order:

- depth of tear — from the fouchette into the greatest depth of the perineal body
- length of tear — from the fouchette into the apex of the vaginal tear
- length of tear — from the fouchette along perineal skin towards the anus.

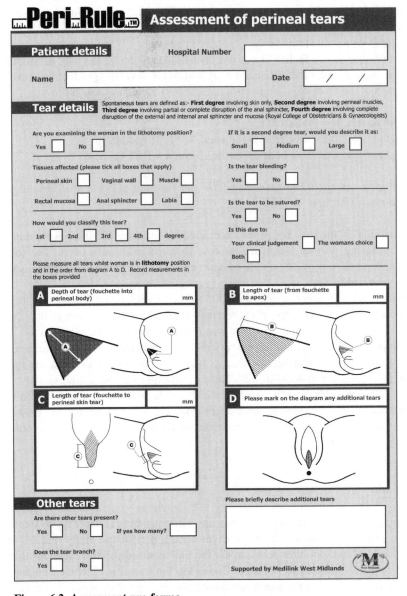

**Figure 6.2: Assessment pro forma**

## Reliability of the Peri-Rule™

A vital piece of the work in developing the Peri-Rule™ was ensuring the reliability of the tool (ie. both the measuring device and the assessment pro forma guiding its use). Measurements needed to be consistent between different midwives otherwise the whole tool would provide unreliable and meaningless data.

The tool was validated by requesting two midwives to measure the tear, the second midwife blinded to the measurements made by the first. It was calculated that to have sufficient statistical power (85% at p<0.05) a total of 130 perineal tears should be assessed with the tool by two midwives (raters). The total number of midwives taking part as first and second rater, however, is unknown because midwives would not sign the research data collection sheet.

The results showed there was a strong level of agreement between the midwife raters to within 5mm of each other (Metcalfe *et al*, 2002). The level of agreement (kappa score, κ) for each of the three measurements using the Peri-Rule™ was as follows:

- depth of tear, $\kappa = 0.67$ (p<0.05)
- length of tear from fouchette to the apex, $\kappa = 0.71$ (p<0.05)
- length of tear from fouchette to perineal skin, $\kappa = 0.75$ (p<0.05)

Note: Kappa scores (κ) greater than 0.61 demonstrate a good level of agreement between raters (Altman, 1991).

The reliability of the tool is further underlined by the fact that there were numerous midwives taking part as raters, across four different maternity units. The tool can therefore be used to provide reliable measurements for simple second-degree tears and is well validated.

Upon originally commencing the pilot work, the tool was also used to attempt to measure the width of the gape of the tear but it quickly became apparent that this was highly subjective and the measurement was removed from the study protocol.

The pro forma currently offers no specific guidelines as to what constitutes a small, medium and large second-degree tear; it merely highlights factors that the midwife may wish to consider in deciding her course of action in the care of individual women. However, the importance of the pro forma is that it provides a mechanism of recording perineal trauma and provides accurate documentation. This will enable the midwives to use the data for future audits and reviews of clinical practice to examine the outcomes of care provision.

## Practicality

The simplicity of the tool and pro forma has made it practical and easy to implement and use in clinical practice. The midwives taking part in the study that led to the development of the tool often learnt to use the tool in simple training sessions that took from five to ten minutes in duration. These teaching sessions included guidance on assessing and measuring the tear using the Peri-Rule™ pro forma as a guide. Teaching sessions were also included in suturing workshops. A CD-ROM providing tuition on the use of the Peri-Rule™ has been developed and this will be included as part of the 'Peri-Rule™ package to maternity units.

## Midwives experiences of using the tool

All the midwives at the teaching sessions understood what measurements were required and agreed that they would simply be measuring what they routinely assessed and did not identify any problems with the pro forma. From anecdotal evidence, the tool was described as easy to use and did not increase workload. Indeed, some midwives reported that it made their assessment of trauma quicker and supported them in making a guided and thorough assessment. Several experienced midwives said that the tool aided their identification of third-degree tears, which they might have previously missed because initial assessment had not revealed the extensiveness of the trauma. This phenomenon is not unique to the Birmingham Perineal Research Evaluation Group study. Other studies on perineal trauma and repair also found that if midwives were asked to carry out a fuller assessment of the perineum following childbirth, the number of third-degree tears identified rose dramatically.

Newly qualified midwives and student midwives particularly liked the tool because it helped them improve their clinical skills and become more confident in assessing perineal trauma.

There were disadvantages and some mixed views regarding the use of the tool to measure perineal tears. This was because some midwives felt that their clinical judgement in assessing the tear and deciding whether the tear should be sutured or left to heal naturally was being questioned. The other drawback was initially the actual measuring device arrived in its own sterile packaging, separate from the main delivery pack. Midwives had to remove their gloves to open the device before using another pair of gloves. This problem is now more easily overcome, as the measuring device can be placed in and sterilised as part of the main delivery pack.

## Women's experiences of the tool

Sustaining a perineal tear during childbirth and needing to have stitches is a concern for many women and all those asked to participate in the early development of the tool agreed. This included a number of women who had previously experienced perineal tears during childbirth. Many were surprised that the tool caused them no discomfort beyond what they were already experiencing from their perineum. Further, no woman complained of increased discomfort from the use of the measuring device. A number of women expressed their support for the use of the device as a more accurate record of the trauma they sustained.

## Benefits of the Peri-Rule™

The reliability of the Peri-Rule™ means that midwives can now measure perineal trauma, providing an excellent resource for education, audit and research on the care of women's perineal trauma following childbirth. For the first time, a standardised approach can be used to measure and document second-degree perineal trauma. Further work is required to develop a severity scale. However, consistent patterns of rated severity began to emerge whilst assessing the reliability of the measuring device (Metcalfe *et al*, 2002), although the numbers were relatively small. Further work is already underway to develop a consensus of opinion between midwives about rating sizes of tears and their level of severity.

## Risk management

The main aim of perineal tear assessment is to support midwives in assessing and diagnosing perineal trauma to reduce the number of women that might endure medium- to long-term complications resulting from undiagnosed tear severity. Assessment will also provide audit and feedback of clinical practice in order that midwives can learn the outcomes of their decision-making. There is also a socio-economic element to the need for better perineal tear assessment. From data provided by the UK NHS Litigation Authority (NHSLA, 2004), since 1 April 1995 there have been 231 claims by women that have sustained perineal trauma following childbirth with a projected cost of £13.5 million pounds, which calculates an average total claim of £58,521 per incident. The NHS has therefore paid an average of £1.5 million pounds per annum in litigation during the last nine years. However, the actual financial costs may be even higher because prior to April 2002, lower value claims were handled internally by NHS Trusts. Unfortunately, from the data collected by the NHSLA, it is not possible to define the information by perineal tear descriptors or whether the litigation was due to a delayed or misdiagnosis of the severity of the perineal trauma. The cost-effectiveness of improving perineal tear assessment may significantly reduce NHS funding lost to litigation. It is worth considering also that the litigation cost figures only reflect the numbers of women that have successfully pursued their claims and do not necessarily include all the costs of the legal process.

The cost not only of litigation but also the number of women that have to return to use NHS services because of problems with the perineum is also considerable. In a recent audit survey of all maternity units in the UK (response rate 82/240, 34%) (unpublished data, Metcalfe and Henderson, 2003), 54% of responding units did not keep records of the number of women returning with problems to the perineum. Of those that did, the numbers of women returning ranged from 0 to 5% of the total number women having a normal vaginal delivery. Four NHS trusts reported that they were in the process of setting up specialist clinics for women that sustained perineal trauma because of the numbers that were experiencing problems. Nine (11%) of the units did not keep data on perineal trauma at all, despite the significant numbers of women involved. (There was an average normal delivery rate for the nine units of 2,026 per year.)

The numbers of women experiencing problems following perineal trauma have been reported to be between 15–20%, but many are reluctant to discuss it with health professionals (Glazener *et al*, 1995, 1997). This suggests there are a large number of women who would benefit from improved assessment of perineal trauma and the subsequent research and audit that needs to take place. The outcomes of such work could have a major impact on the physical and psychological health of many childbearing women.

The Peri-Rule™ provides an opportunity to collate objective perineal tear measurements which can be used to develop audits of practice, to highlight any possible problems or difficulties with procedures or guidelines. The relatively small financial outlay of purchasing the Peri-Rule™ and encouraging midwives to use the tool to improve the assessment of perineal trauma is likely to lead to significantly fewer cases of litigation, which could prove extremely cost-effective, especially as during the validation of the Peri-Rule's reliability, some midwives reported that they had found third degree perineal trauma requiring medical intervention. Upon their initial assessments of the perineal trauma, the midwives had thought that the tear had appeared to be more superficial.

## The international perspective

Internationally, several groups have expressed an interest in using the Peri-Rule™ as a means of assessing perineal trauma following childbirth, including developed and developing countries. However, in developing countries there are additional issues relating to the importance of perineal trauma, as referred to in *Chapter 2*.

High levels of maternal morbidity and mortality observed in many developing countries is related to a complex range of inter-related health problems However, perineal trauma and its poor assessment is one of the related problems which often results in infection leading to morbidity and mortality for many women. Many women live in remote areas, several hundreds of miles away from hospital or medical care. (UNICEF, 1999) Further, as highlighted in *Chapter 1*, many do not have access to a trained midwife. Improvements in being able to offer guidelines on the assessment of perineal trauma to midwives or health support workers in more remote areas, would enable them to make a more robust assessment and supported judgements in seeking further medical care for more severe types of perineal trauma. Such supported decision-making can be crucial in deciding whether to transport women to receive further medical treatment for their perineal tears. In addition, the accumulation of data in poorer countries could assist UNICEF (United Nations Children's Fund) and WHO (World Health Organization) to push for reform and prioritisation of health services provision in these poorer countries.

## Future work

In validating the tool, the midwife raters were asked only to measure and record single tears. The tool is being developed further to measure more complex and branched tears which will include methods of annotating descriptions of all different types of perineal trauma.

Work is already underway to develop a severity rating based upon size of second-degree tear and whether the sizes of different anatomical features of the perineum are likely to increase or reduce the risk of perineal trauma. For example, does the distance between fourchette and anal margin make a difference as to the type of perineal trauma that is likely to be sustained? There is also the opportunity to discuss further the potential of undertaking randomised controlled trial comparing the effectiveness of suturing versus non-suturing following the development of a reliable tool to assess and compare size of trauma.

## Conclusion

The Peri-Rule™ assessment provides the first pragmatic method of collecting baseline data that can be used to inform audit and research which, in turn, inform clinical practice to improve care of perineal trauma. Particularly, second-degree perineal tears, where there can be such a large variation in size and there is disagreement on the most appropriate treatment. For the first time information can be collated which can provide evidence on the outcomes of different types of care for perineal wound care based on objective measurement and comparison of tear sizes.

The major benefit of the Peri-Rule™ is its simplicity. The measuring device is simple and quick to use, causing minimal discomfort to women undergoing assessment. It also assists midwives themselves because the tool takes just a few seconds to use and the assessment pro forma guides each stage of the evaluation of the trauma. Its aim is to support midwives clinical decision-making rather than remove it. In addition, other benefits of the tool also emerged that are particularly important to women's health outcomes following perineal trauma. Midwives found that by using the tool for assessment of tears encouraged closer examination of the perineum, which improved the diagnosis of more severe trauma.

Further work is underway to develop the pro forma for the assessment of more complex tears and it is hoped to develop a severity scale. The Peri-Rule™ also offers the opportunity to develop the much needed randomised controlled trial to compare suturing versus non-suturing of second-degree tears as, for the first time, there is a reliable, pragmatic method of measuring and comparing size of second-degree perineal trauma.

# References

Altman D G (1991) *Practical Statistics for Medical Research*. Chapman and Hall, London

Clement S, Reed B (1999) To stitch or not to stitch. A long term follow up study of women with unsutured perineal tears. *Practice Midwife* **2**(4): 20–8

Davidson NS (1974) REEDA evaluating postpartum healing. *J Nurse-Midwifery* **19**: 6–9

Glazener CMA, Abdalla M, Stroud P, Naji S, Templeton A, Russell IT (1995) Postnatal maternal morbidity: extent, causes, prevention and treatment. *Br J Obstet Gynaecol* **102**(4): 282–7

Glazener CMA (1997) Sexual function after childbirth: women's experiences, persistent morbidity and lack of professional recognition. *Br J Obstet Gynaecol* **104**(3): 330–5

Gomme C, Yiannouzis K, Ullman R (2001) Developing a tool to assess perineal trauma. *Br J Midwif* **9**(9): 538–44

Head M (1993) Dropping stitches. *Nurs Times* **89**(33): 64–5

Hill, P (1990) Psychometric properties of the REEDA. *J Nurse-Midwifery* **35**(3): 162–5

Metcalfe AM, Tohill S, Williams A, Haldon V, Brown L, Henry L (2002) A pragmatic tool for the measurement of perineal tears. *Br J Midwifery* **10**(7): 412–17

Metcalfe AM, Henderson C (2003) *Audit Survey of Maternity Units in the UK*. Unpublished.

NHS Litigation Authority (2004) Personal email communication. NHSLA, March

Royal College of Obstetrics and Gynaecology (2004) Clinical Green Top Guidelines-Perineal Repair. Methods and Material used in Perineal Repair(23). Online at: http://www.rcog.org.uk/print.asp?PageID=106&Type=guidelines&GuidelineID=15 (accessed 18 February 2004)

Steen M, Cooper K (1997) A tool for assessing perineal trauma. *J Wound Care* **6**(9): 432–6

Ullman RM, Yiannouzis K, Gomme CC (2004) Testing a tool to assess perineal trauma. *Br J Midwifery* **12**(2): 93–100

UNICEF (1999) Online at: http://www.unicef.org/pon96/woestima.htm. (accessed 1 March 2004)

# 7

## Prevention of obstetric perineal trauma

*Ranee Thakar and Abdul Sultan*

### Introduction

Obstetric perineal trauma is a cause of significant morbidity that can have a dramatic effect on women's quality of life. Unfortunately, it is under-reported as many women suffer in silence (Glazener *et al*, 1995). Perineal trauma can occur spontaneously or intentionally by a surgical incision (episiotomy). It is estimated that over 85% of women who have spontaneous vaginal birth will sustain some form of perineal trauma and of these 60–70% will require suturing (Sleep *et al*, 1984; McCandlish *et al*, 1998). There are international variations in episiotomy rates as described in *Chapter 5*. Variations are also dependent on birth attendant (Henriksen *et al*, 1994; Klein *et al*, 1994) and hospital practice (Rockner and Olund, 1991). As Graham and Davies describe in *Chapter 5*, the fall in episiotomy rates in the United Kingdom, The United States and other countries has been attributed to prominent consumer advocacy, a force not yet effectively engaged in this area in many other countries, where professionals remain dominant.

Recognised anal sphincter rupture is reported in about 2.5% of vaginal deliveries in centres that practise mediolateral episiotomy and up to 19% in centres that practise midline episiotomy (Sultan, 1997; Fenner *et al*, 2003). However, 33% of women sustain 'occult' anal sphincter injury (ie. defects in the anal sphincter detected by anal endosonography) following vaginal delivery (Sultan *et al*, 1993). The most plausible explanation for an 'occult' injury is either an injury that has been missed, recognised but not reported or wrongly classified as a second degree tear (Thakar and Sultan, 2003). As a result of inconsistency in classification and under-reporting of perineal trauma, it is difficult to establish the true global incidence of perineal trauma.

Perineal trauma can be associated with considerable short and long-term morbidity as highlighted in *Chapter 8*: perineal pain can occur in up to 42% of women ten to twelve days postpartum and about 10% will continue to suffer in the long term; 23% reported dyspareunia at three months, 10% anal incontinence and 19% urinary incontinence (RCOG guideline No 23, 2003). Other complications include perineal infection, fistulae and endometriosis of perineal wounds. Maternal activity and infant feeding may also be affected. Preventing even some childbirth trauma would benefit a large number of women. It would also result both in cost savings (by reducing the amount of drugs, suturing and treatments needed), and time spent by caregivers helping new mothers deal with the aftermath of this trauma.

Although the case for prevention of perineal trauma is compelling, how to accomplish this is less clear. Certain antenatal risk factors, such as maternal nutritional status, body mass index, ethnicity, infant birth weight (Renfrew *et al*, 1998), race and age (Howard *et al*, 2000) cannot be altered at birth but their presence might prompt modifications in the care pathway. Factors that are under the control of the birth attendant are episiotomy, previous perineal tears, instrumental deliveries, maternal positions, fetal malpositions delivery methods and pushing technique.

Preventative strategies can be instituted at three levels. Primary prevention involves preventing disease from occurring by removing its causes. Secondary prevention strategies would involve detecting a disease early and treating it to stop progression. Tertiary preventative strategies would involve activities that prevent deterioration or reduce complications after a disease has declared itself.

In this chapter, we intend to use these definitions to discuss the preventative measures that can be taken to reduce perineal trauma. The data have been obtained from a combination of references from the electronic MEDLINE (1966–2004) and those obtained through a hand-search of the citations revealed by the initial electronic search. Where relevant, text books and personal experience are quoted.

## Primary prevention strategies

### Elective caesarean section

Elective caesarean section is the only form of delivery that can totally ensure absence of perineal trauma. However, compared to vaginal delivery, caesarean section is associated with an increased mortality (three-fold increase in UK) even when it is performed as an elective procedure (Hall and Bewley, 1999). Maternal morbidity is also increased, in addition to risk of complications associated with any other major abdominal surgery (Sultan and Stanton, 1996), the risk of a caesarean hysterectomy as a life-saving procedure is increased by more than ten-fold. Clark *et al* (1985) reviewed almost 100,000 deliveries and noted that the risk of placenta praevia increased linearly with the number of previous caesarean sections and rose to 10% in women with four or more caesarean sections. The risk of placenta accreta in these women also increased to as high as 67% after four caesarean sections. Overall, the risk of caesarean hysterectomy due to placenta accreta following a previous caesarean section was 72%. Caesarean hysterectomy, in turn, is also associated with an increased morbidity and mortality. Furthermore, a caesarean section performed solely to prevent perineal trauma will be a recurrent indication in subsequent pregnancies and therefore cumulative mortality and morbidity should always be considered.

Currently, prophylactic elective caesarean section is being promoted to prevent incontinence but without robust evidence. Elective caesarean section has been suggested to be protective (MacArthur *et al*, 2001; Sultan *et al*, 1993; Fynes *et al*, 1998). Fynes *et al* (1998) followed 234 women (200 spontaneous delivery and thirty-four caesarean sections) and found that after vaginal delivery 19% developed anal incontinence and 33% had evidence of anal sphincter injury. Women who delivered by caesarean section did not develop anal incontinence and there was no evidence of anal sphincter trauma regardless of the stage of labour. However, when caesarean section was performed after the cervix had dilated to more than 8 cm there was a reduction in anal squeeze pressure increment and pudendal nerve terminal motor latencies were prolonged. Sultan *et al* (1994a) also reported a similar phenomenon when caesarean section was performed after prolonged labour and engagement of the head. The long-term implication of this finding remains to be established. In a retrospective comparative study, looking at incidence and severity of anal incontinence in primiparae after caesarean (104 emergency and 80 elective) with those who had a non-instrumental vaginal delivery (n=100), Lal *et al* (2003) found that elective caesarean or pre-labour emergency caesarean is not always protective, and symptoms of incontinence maybe severe, suggesting that pregnancy itself can lead to pelvic floor dysfunction. Further, prospective studies need to be performed to investigate this issue.

## Secondary prevention strategies

### Episiotomy

Episiotomy is the surgical enlargement of the vaginal orifice by an incision of the perineum during the last part of the second stage of labour to enlarge the vaginal orifice. Although there is a lack of scientific evidence regarding its effectiveness (Thacker and Banta, 1983; Wooley, 1995) it is still the commonest operation requiring repair in obstetrics, as described in *Chapter 5*.

A Cochrane review including six studies designed to evaluate the benefits of episiotomy reveals that compared with routine use, restrictive episiotomy involved less posterior perineal trauma, less suturing and fewer healing complications. The only disadvantage of restrictive episiotomy was an increased risk of anterior perineal trauma. There was no difference in severe vaginal or perineal trauma; dyspareunia, urinary incontinence or several pain measures (Carroli and Belizan, 2004). This suggests that the practice of routine episiotomy is obsolete and has no place in modern obstetrics.

The question of whether midline episiotomy results in better outcome than mediolateral episiotomy has not been satisfactorily answered (Carroli and Belizan, 2004). Midline episiotomies are more popular in North America as it is believed that they are more comfortable and recovery is less complicated. However, Coats *et al* (1980) performed a randomised study of 407 primiparae and found 12% of midline episiotomies extended into the anal sphincter compared to 2% of mediolateral episiotomies. Although the perineum was significantly less bruised in the midline group and sexual intercourse commenced earlier, pain and wound breakdown was similar in both groups. The results of this study must be viewed with caution as allocation to this study was quasi random and therefore prone to bias. In addition, when an incision was inappropriate to the treatment allocation, the woman was removed from the trial. This increased the risk of selection bias as analysis was not performed according to 'intention to treat'. However, some retrospective studies have shown that mediolateral episiotomy may protect against obstetric anal sphincter injury (Poen *et al*, 1997; Anthony *et al*, 1994; DeLeeuw *et al*, 2001), while others have described a strong association with midline episiotomy (Bodner-Adler *et al*, 2001; Fenner *et al*, 2003; Klein *et al*, 1994; Shiono *et al*, 1990).

## Previous perineal trauma

In centres that practise midline episiotomy, a previous third or fourth degree tear is a risk factor for a repeat third/fourth degree tear (Payne *et al*, 1999; Peleg *et al*, 1999). In a large retrospective study of 1895 women, Martin *et al* (2001) found that having perineal trauma at the first delivery more than tripled the risk of spontaneous tears at second delivery. The risk of spontaneous tears at second delivery increased depending on the severity of the previous perineal trauma at the first delivery.

## Instrumental delivery

Although only 4% of women delivered by forceps sustain a third/fourth degree tear, up to 50% of those that do tear had a forceps delivery (Sultan *et al*, 1994b). Compared to forceps delivery, vacuum extraction is associated with fewer third/fourth degree tears and this view is supported by two large randomised studies (Bofill *et al*, 1996; Johanson *et al*, 1993). A UK study (Johanson *et al*, 1993) where mediolateral episiotomy is practised, reported severe vaginal lacerations in 17% of forceps compared to 11% of vacuum deliveries and a Canadian study (Bofill *et al*, 1993) where midline episiotomy is practised reported third/fourth degree tears in 29% of forceps compared to 12% of vacuum deliveries. In a Cochrane review of ten trials (Johanson and Menon, 2004) use of the vacuum extractor instead of forceps was associated with significantly less maternal trauma and with less need for general and regional anaesthesia. There were more deliveries with vacuum extraction and fewer caesarean sections were carried out in the vacuum extractor group. However, the vacuum extractor was associated with an increase in neonatal cephalhaematomata and retinal haemorrhages. Serious neonatal injury was uncommon with either instrument. A five-year follow-up of infants who participated in a randomised study of forceps and vacuum delivery has confirmed that there is no difference in terms of neurological development and visual acuity with use of either instrument (Johanson *et al*, 1999). Occult trauma to the anal sphincter has also been identified more frequently in forceps delivery occurring in up to 80 per cent of women (Sultan *et al*, 1998). Trauma occurs more frequently when a second instrument is used to attempt vaginal delivery (Sultan *et al*, 1998) and therefore if delivery fails with the appropriate technique and vacuum cup, one should resort to a caesarean section. Metal cups appear to be more suitable for 'occipito-posterior', transverse and difficult 'occipito-anterior' position deliveries (Johanson and Menon, 2004). The soft cups seem to be appropriate for straightforward deliveries as they are significantly more likely to fail to achieve vaginal delivery. Although they were associated with less scalp injury, there was no difference between the two groups in terms of maternal injury. Farrell *et al* (2001) performed a prospective study of 690 primigravid women and found that forceps delivery was associated with a higher incidence of flatus incontinence compared to vaginal delivery and both flatus and faecal incontinence compared to caesarean delivery. Vacuum delivery did not increase the risk of flatus incontinence. MacArthur *et al* (2001) performed the largest questionnaire based multicentre study and reported a 9.2% prevalence of faecal incontinence at three months post-partum. Compared to vacuum extraction, forceps delivery was associated with almost twice the risk of developing faecal incontinence. These studies support the recommendation by the Royal College of Obstetricians and Gynaecologists that the vacuum extractor should be the instrument of choice (RCOG, 1993).

## Delivery position

It has been postulated that position at delivery (upright or lying down) may influence the risk of perineal trauma. However, the Cochrane review (Gupta and Nikodem, 2004) has shown that with the possible exception of increased blood loss (>500 mls), no deleterious effects have been demonstrated to the mother or fetus with delivery in the upright posture. The current evidence on the effectiveness of various delivery positions remains inconclusive.

## Delivery techniques

Pirhonen *et al* (1998) compared the frequency of anal sphincter rupture in low risk deliveries between two Scandinavian countries (26 541 vaginal deliveries) and found the risk to be thirteen times higher in Sweden (Malmo) vs Finland (Turku). They speculated that the only explanation for this was a difference in manual support given to the baby's head during crowning and pushing the perineum under the chin.

Traditionally, manual support of the perineum has been regarded as mandatory for protecting maternal tissue during delivery. It is widely believed that guarding the perineum during delivery of the fetal head prevents or reduces perineal trauma. The National Perinatal Epidemiological Unit at Oxford conducted a randomised controlled trial of hands on or poised (HOOP) methods of delivery (McCandlish *et al*, 1998). At the end of second stage of labour women were allocated to either 'hands on' (the midwife's hands put pressure on the baby's head and support the perineum; lateral flexion is then used to facilitate the delivery of the shoulders) or the 'hands poised' (the midwife keeps her hands poised, not touching the head or perineum, allowing spontaneous delivery of the shoulders). They found that a reduction in pain at ten days was noted in the 'hands on' group (31.1% versus 34.1%, p=0.02), but the rate of episiotomy was significantly lower in the 'hands poised' group. However, 30% of the hands poised group converted to the hands on after randomization and analysis was based on intention to treat. Mayerhofer *et al* (2002) in another similar randomised study using perineal trauma as a primary outcome measure found that women receiving hands on care had a significantly higher rate of third degree perineal tears (2.7% versus 0.9%). Likewise, the episiotomy rate was significantly higher in the hands on group (17.9% versus 10.1%), but there was no statistically significant difference in overall perineal trauma between the two groups.

## Malposition

The incidence of persistent occipito-posterior (OP) position of the fetal head varies between 1 to 5% and it has been identified as a risk factor for perineal trauma (Sultan *et al*, 1994b; Fitzpatrick *et al*, 2000), presumably due to the greater cephalic diameter presenting to the perineum. Fitzpatrick *et al* compared 246 women with persistent OP position in labour compared to 13,543 contemporaneous vaginal deliveries with occipito-anterior (OA) position. Compared to the OA group, obstetric anal sphincter trauma was significantly more common in the OP group (7% versus 1%) irrespective of parity. The incidence of episiotomy (mediolateral) was similar (85% in OP group 76% in OA group). Persistent OP position was also associated with prolonged labour and instrumental delivery in both primiparous and multiparous women. Although epidural use was also significantly higher in the OP position, they suggested that this was an association rather than a cause of the OP position as substantial increase in epidural use over the years in their institution has not increased the frequency of OP position. It has been suggested that use of epidural after engagement of the fetal head is associated with decrease in incidence of OP position (Robinson *et al*, 1996). Other methods of preventing OP position at delivery are manual or instrumental rotation of the head to OA and the use of syntocinon.

## Prolonged second stage of labour

Donnelly *et al* (1998) reported that instrumental vaginal delivery and a passive second stage of labour prolonged by epidural analgesia were significantly associated with the risk of anal sphincter trauma and impaired faecal continence. As instrumental delivery is a known risk factor (eight-fold increased risk of sphincter trauma), early use of oxytocin was recommended to shorten the second stage.

## Epidural analgesia

There are conflicting data on the effect of epidural analgesia on perineal trauma. Robinson *et al* (1999) showed that women who had epidural analgesia were more likely to have perineal trauma, but this was due to the increased operative vaginal deliveries and episiotomies with epidurals. Poen *et al* (1997) found an increased risk of anal sphincter injury due to epidural and suggested that this could be due to relief of pain which normally functions as an alarm for perineal stretching. In contrast, Combs *et al* (1990) suggest that relaxation of perineal musculature prevents women from having anal sphincter tears during instrumental delivery. Others have found a significant increase in episiotomy rate during vaginal delivery with an epidural but without an increase in perineal tears (Bodner-Adler *et al*, 2002). Overall, it appears that the increased perineal trauma is related to the associated increase in instrumental delivery (Lieberman and O'Donoghue, 2002).

## Pushing methods

Fraser *et al* (2000) randomised 1862 nulliparous women at the time of full dilatation to either a delayed pushing (advised to wait at least two hours after full dilatation) or early pushing (commence as soon as randomised). The aim was to determine whether a policy of delayed pushing with epidural analgesia would reduce the risk of difficult delivery (defined as caesarean section, operative delivery or low pelvic procedure with rotation greater than forty-five degrees). Delayed pushing was associated with a reduction in difficult deliveries compared with early pushing after controlling for duration of first stage of labour and station of fetal head at randomisation. The frequency of episiotomy and third and fourth degree tears did not differ in the two groups because delayed pushing did not reduce the number of difficult deliveries sufficiently to produce better perineal outcome. Fitzpatrick *et al* (2002) confirmed these findings and, in addition, found that the instrumental delivery rates, anal incontinence, anal manometry and ultrasound neurophysiology studies did not differ between the two groups.

## Identification and repair of third degree tears

The underlying pathophysiology behind anal sphincter trauma is complex and includes neurological and mechanical factors, which can lead to anal incontinence. Until the advent of anal endosonography, anal incontinence was largely attributed to neurogenic trauma. We reviewed the English literature since 1980 and found twenty studies reporting anal incontinence ranging between 15 to 59% following immediate repair of obstetric anal sphincter rupture (Sultan and Thakar, 2002). The mean prevalence of anal incontinence was 37%. However, frank faecal incontinence affected 9% (range 2 to 23%). Using anal endosonography persistent anal sphincter defects following repair were identified in 40 to 91% of women (Sultan and Thakar, 2002). Although end-to-end approximation was most popular, the actual technique was not always described. Colorectal surgeons prefer the overlap technique for patients presenting with faecal incontinence although longer-term follow-up suggests that symptoms may deteriorate with time. Based on this, Sultan *et al* (1999) described that the overlap technique for the external sphincter and separate approximation of the internal sphincter. Although they obtained very favourable results with the overlap technique it could be a reflection of operator expertise and therefore they recommended a randomised study. There is only one published randomised trial to date by Fitzpatrick *et al* (2000) in which 112 primiparous women were recruited. No significant difference between the two methods of repair were identified, although there appeared to be a trend towards more symptoms in the end-to-end group. Compared to Sultan's description (Sultan *et al*, 1999) there were methodological differences in that the torn internal sphincter was not identified and repaired separately and they used a constipating agent for three days after the repair. It is also unclear as to how overlap was performed in women who had partial tears of the external sphincter. Nevertheless, as the authors concur, a better outcome would be expected with both techniques as a consequence of focused education and training in anal sphincter repair. A longer-term follow-up is awaited and further randomised trials using the described technique are currently in progress. However, the evidence to date indicates that there is no significant difference in short-term outcome with the end-to-end or overlap technique and either technique can be used.

We have recently shown that 90% of third degree tears are being missed by midwives (Andrews *et al*, 2004). Furthermore, more than two thirds of doctors practising obstetrics feel inadequately trained in perineal anatomy and repair. It is imperative that more focused training is intensified. In this regard, Thakar *et al* have introduced an ongoing course using video presentations, specially designed models and fresh animal anorectal specimens to demonstrate anatomy and techniques of repair (www.perineum. net). The feedback from attendees is that this type of training has resulted in a change in practice and should become an essential part of the modular training for specialist registrars (Thakar *et al*, 2001).

## Ancillary methods

### *Perineal massage*

Stretching and massaging of the perineum in the antenatal period and during the second stage of labour has been promoted as a means of increasing the elasticity of the perineum and reducing the need for episiotomy. The protective value of perineal massage during the antenatal period has been evaluated in two randomised studies. It involves digital perineal stretching, with oil lubrication from thirty-five weeks gestation for about ten minutes everyday. In the United Kingdom, Shipman *et al* (1997) randomised 861 nulliparous women and found a non-significant benefit of 6% in the prevalence of perineal trauma (75% versus 69%,P<0.07), but a secondary analysis by maternal age, showed a much larger benefit (12.1%) with massage among those aged thirty years and over. In a larger randomised study, Labrecque *et al* (1999) found that among participants without a previous vaginal birth, a significantly greater number of women in the experimental group (24%) delivered with an intact perineum compared to the control group (15%). A dose-response effect was observed. However, for women who had a previous vaginal delivery, there were no differences in intact perineum rates between the experimental and control groups. This effect means that for every ten women doing perineal massage there will be one additional woman whose perineum remains intact after delivery. More importantly, pregnant women find perineal massage acceptable. This study is encouraging in demonstrating the effectiveness of a simple, woman controlled intervention to maintain perineal integrity. At three months postpartum, there was no difference in perineal function between women who had and those that had not received perineal massage (Labrecque *et al*, 2000).

Perineal massage has also been advocated in the second stage of labour, which is provided by the midwife by inserting two fingers in the vagina, and using a sweeping motion, to stretch the perineum with lubricating gel with each uterine contraction. In a randomised study, Stamp *et al* (2001) found no benefit from massage in terms of an intact perineum or pain.

Available evidence suggests that perineal massage may be beneficial to mothers if performed during the antenatal period, especially if they have not had a previous vaginal delivery. Although perineal massage in labour does not increase the likelihood of an intact perineum, it is a harmless practice and midwives can follow their usual practice while taking into account the preferences of the woman.

## Water births

Anecdotal reports suggest that the perineum is more pliable in water and can stretch more easily, resulting in less trauma. However, a recent Cochrane review (Cluett *et al*, 2004) showed no difference in episiotomy or perineal tears after immersion in water during first and second stage. However, there is evidence that water immersion during the first stage of labour reduces the use of analgesia and maternal pain, without adverse outcomes on labour duration, operative delivery or neonatal outcomes.

## Home birth

In a prospective observational study of 1068 women, Murphy and Feinland (1998) looked at perineal outcomes in a home birth setting. In this sample, 69.6% had an intact perineum, 1.4% had an episiotomy, 29% had a first or second degree tear and 0.7% had obstetric anal sphincter injury. Logistic regression analysis showed that in multiparas, low socioeconomic status and higher parity were associated with intact perineum, whereas increased age (≥40years), previous episiotomy, weight gain over forty pounds, prolonged second stage and the use of oils and lubricants were associated with perineal trauma. Amongst nulliparas, low socioeconomic status, kneeling or hands-and-knees position at delivery, and manual support of the perineum at delivery were associated with an intact perineum, whereas perineal massage during delivery was associated with perineal trauma. The results of this study suggest that it is possible for midwives to achieve a high rate of intact perineums and low rate of episiotomy in a selected setting and population group.

## Tertiary prevention strategies

It is recommended that women who previously had a successful secondary anal sphincter repair for faecal incontinence should be delivered by caesarean section (Sultan and Stanton, 1996). However, the risk:benefit assessment is less clear in an asymptomatic woman with a previous third/fourth degree tear and there are no randomised trials. The risk of recurrence of such tears is very low (less than 5%) and caution should be exercised before introducing a recurrent indication for caesarean section with its attendant morbidity and mortality.

Women should be followed up in hospital by an experienced obstetrician six to eight weeks after delivery. As described in *Chapter 8*, some centres have dedicated multidisciplinary perineal clinics. A careful history must be elicited from the patient with information pertaining to bladder, bowel and sexual function being emphasised.

Women should have a careful vaginal and rectal examination to ensure complete healing, and check anal tone and scar tenderness. Ideally, all women should also have anal endosonography (*Figure 7.1*) and manometry. If these facilities are not readily available at least women who are symptomatic should be referred.

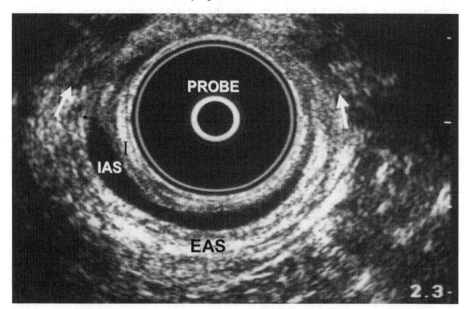

**Figure 7.1: Endoanal scan demonstrating a large defect between 9 and 3 o'clock (between arrows) of the external (EAS) and internal (IAS) anal sphincter (Andrew *et al*, 2003)**

If one is contemplating a vaginal delivery these tests should be perfomed antenatally unless they have been done previously and were abnormal. If the size of defect on ultrasound is greater than one quadrant or if the squeeze pressure increment is less than 20mmHg there is an increased risk of impaired continence (75% vs 5%) following a subsequent delivery (Fynes *et al*, 1999). Such women should be counselled and especially if they have mild symptoms of incontinence (faecal urgency or flatus incontinence) they should be offered a caesarean section. Asymptomatic women who are symptom free can be delivered vaginally by an experienced accoucheur. Prophylactic episiotomy has been practised by some although there is no evidence that it prevents anal sphincter injury and therefore we do not perform episiotomies routinely (Sultan and Thakar, 2002; Andrews *et al*, 2003) (*Figure 7.2*).

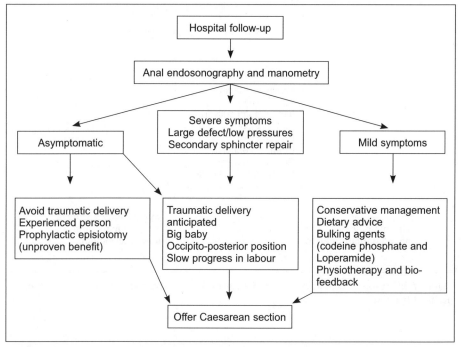

**Figure 7.2: Flow diagram to demonstrate pathway in management of acute obstetric sphincter injury (Andrews *et al*, 2003)**

Women who have severe incontinence following a third or fourth degree tear should have a secondary sphincter repair by a colorectal surgeon and offered a caesarean section for all subsequent deliveries. However, if women want to complete their family prior to secondary sphincter repair it can be argued that women can deliver vaginally as the damage had already occurred.

## Conclusions

World-wide, obstetric perineal trauma can have a devastating effect on a woman's social life with associated psychological sequelae. Consequently, every attempt should be made to prevent such trauma leading to short-term effects such as pain and dyspareunia, or longer-term effects such as prolapse and incontinence. We have highlighted factors in obstetric practice that may be modified to minimise perineal trauma (*Figure 7.3*). It is equally important to recognise and repair trauma appropriately and therefore a focused and intensive training program for doctors and midwives should be essential (Sultan and Thakar, 2003). While caesarean section may eradicate perineal trauma, it is associated with an increased risk of mortality and morbidity and should only be offered selectively (Sultan and Stanton, 1996).

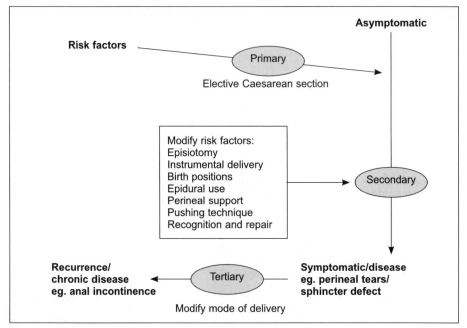

**Figure 7.3: Primary, secondary and tertiary preventative strategies to minimise risk of perineal trauma**

# References

Andrews V, Thakar R, Sultan AH (2003) Management of third and fourth degree tears. *Rev Gynae Pract* **3**: 188–95

Andrews V, Thakar R, Sultan AH (2004) Are midwives adequately trained to identify anal sphincter injury? International Continence Society UK Proceedings. 11th Annual Scientific Meeting: 34

Anthony S, Buitendijk SE, Zondervan KT, van Rijssel EJC, Verkerk PH (1994) Episiotomies and the occurrence of severe perineal lacerations. *Br J Obstet Gynaecol* **101**: 1064–67

Bofill JA, Rust OA, Schorr SJ *et al* (1996) A randomized prospective trial of the obstetric forceps versus the M-cup vacuum extractor. *Am J Obstet Gynecol* **175**: 1325–30

Bodner-Adler B, Bodner K, Kimberger O, Wagenbichler P, Kaider A, Husslein P, Mayerhofer K (2002) The effect of epidural analgesia on the occurrence of obstetric lacerations and on the neonatal outcome during spontaneous vaginal delivery. *Arch Gynecol Obstet* **267**: 81–4

Bodner-Adler B, Bodner K, Kaider A, Wagenbichler P, Leodolter S, Husslein P, Mayerhofer K (2001) Risk factors for third degree perineal tears in vaginal delivery, with an analysis of episiotomy sites. *J Reprod Med* **46**: 752–56

Carroli G, Belizan J (2004) *Episiotomy for vaginal birth*. The Cochrane Library 2004 Issue 4. John Wiley & Sons Ltd, Chichester, UK

Clark SL, Koonings PP, Phelan JP (1985) Placenta praevia,baccreta and prior cesarean section. *Obstet Gynecol* **89**: 89–92

Cluett E R, Nikodem VC, McCandlish RE, Burns EE (2004) Immersion in water in pregnancy, labour and birth (Cochrane Review). In: The Cochrane Library, Issue 2. John Wiley & Sons Ltd, Chichester

Coats PM, Chan KK, Wilkins M, Beard RJ (1980) A comparison between midline and mediolateral episiotomies. *Br J Obstet Gynaecol* **87**: 408–12

Combs CA, Robertson PA, Laros RK Jr (1990) Risk factors for third-degree perineal lacerations in forceps and vacuum deliveries. *Am J Obstet Gynecol* **163**: 100–104

DeLeeuw JW, Vierhout ME, Struijk PC, Wim WCJ, Wallenburg HCS (2001) Anal sphincter injury after vaginal delivery: functional outcome and risk factors for fecal incontinence. *Acta Obstet Gynecol Scand* **80**: 830–34

Donnelly V, Fynes M, Campbell D, Johnson H, O'Connell R, O'Herlihy C (1998) Obstetric events leading to anal sphincter damage. *Obstet Gynecol* **92**: 955–61

Farrell SA, Allen VM, Baskett TF (2001) Anal incontinence in primiparas. *J Soc Obstet Gynaecol Can* **23**: 321–26

Fenner DE, Genberg B, Brahma P, Marek L, DeLancey JOL (2003) Fecal and urinary incontinence after vaginal delivery with anal sphincter disruption in an obstetrics unit in the United States. *Am J Obstet Gynecol* **189**(6): 1543–50

Fitzpatrick M, Behan M, O'Connell R, O'Herlihy C (2000) A randomized clinical trial comparing primary overlap with approximation repair of third-degree obstetric tears. *Am J Obstet Gynecol* **183**: 1220–24

Fitzpatrick M, McQuillan K, O'Herlihy C (2000) Influence of Occipto-posterior position on delivery outcome. *Am J Obstet Gynecol* **182**(1, Part 2): S134

Fitzpatrick M, Harkin R, McQuillan K, O'Brien C, O'Connell PR, O'Herlihy (2002) A randomised clinical trial comparing the effects of delayed versus immediate pushing with epidural analgesia on mode of delivery and faecal incontinence. *Br J Obstet Gynaecol* **109**: 1359–65

Fynes M, Donnelly V, Behan M, O'Connell PR, O'Herlihy C (1999) Effect of second vaginal delivery on anorectal physiology and faecal incontinence: a prospective study. *Lancet* **354**: 983–6

Fynes M, Donelly VS, O'Connell PR, O'Herlihy C (1998) Caesarean delivery and anal sphincter injury. *Obstet Gynecol* **92**: 496–500

Fraser WD, Marcoux S, Krauss I, Douglas J, Goulet C, Boulvain M (2000) Multicenter, randomised trial, controlled trial of delayed pushing for nulliparous women in second stage of labor with continuous epidural. *Am J Obstet Gynecol* **182**: 1165–72

Glazener CMA, Abdalla M, Stroud P, Naji S, Templeton A, Russell IT (1995) Postnatal maternal morbidity: extent, causes, prevention and treatment. *Br J Obstet Gynaecol* **102**: 282–7

Graham ID (1997) *Episiotomy: challenging interventions*. Blackwell Science, Oxford

Gupta JK , Nikodem VC (2004) Woman's position during second stage of labour (Cochrane Review). In: The Cochrane Library, Issue 4. Update Software, Oxford

Hall MH, Bewley S (1999) Maternal mortality and mode of delivery. *Lancet* **354**: 776

Henriksen TB, Bek KM, Hedegaard M, Secher NJ (1994) Methods and consequences of changes in use of episiotomy. *Br Med J* **309**: 1255–8

Howard D, Davies PS, Delancey JOL, Small Yvonne (2000) Differences in perineal lacerations in black and white primiparas. *Obstet Gynecol* **96**: 622–24

Johanson RB, Heycock E, Carter J, Sultan AH, Walklate K, Jones PW (1999) Maternal and child health after assisted vaginal delivery: five-year follow up of a randomised controlled study comparing forceps and ventouse. *Br J Obstet Gynaecol* **106**: 544–49

Johanson RB, Menon BKV (2001) Soft versus rigid vacuum extractor cups for assisted vaginal delivery; Vacuum extraction versus forceps for assisted vaginal delivery. In: The Cochrane Library, Issue 1. Update Software, Oxford

Johanson RB, Menon BKV (2004) Vacuum extraction versus forceps for assisted vaginal delivery (Cochrane Review). In: The Cochrane Library, Issue 4. Update Software, Oxford

Johanson RB, Rice C, Doyle M *et al* (1993) A randomised prospective study comparing the new vacuum extractor policy with forceps delivery. *Br J Obstet Gynaecol* **100**: 524–30

Kettle C, Johanson RB (2001) Continuous versus interrupted sutures for perineal repair (Cochrane Review). In: The Cochrane Library, Issue 2. Update Software, Oxford

Klein MC, Gauthier RJ, Robbins JG, Kaczorowski J, Jorgenesen SH, Franco ED *et al* (1994) Relationship of episiotomy to perineal trauma and morbidity, sexual dysfunction, and pelvic floor relaxation. *Am J Obstet Gynecol* **171**: 591–98

Labrecque M, Eason E, Marcoux S *et al* (1999) Randomised controlled trial of prevention of perineal trauma by perineal massage during pregnancy. *Am J Obstet Gynecol* **180**: 593–600

Labrecque M, Eason E, Marcoux S (2000) Randomized controlled trial of prevention of perineal trauma by perineal massage during pregnancy. *Am J Obstet Gynecol* **182**: 76–80

Lal M, Mann CH, Callender R, Radley S (2003) Does caesarean delivery prevent anal incontinence? *Obstet Gynecol* **101**: 305–12

Lieberman E, ODonoghue C (2002) Unintended effects of epidural analgesia during labor: A systematic review. *Am J Obstet Gynecol* **186**: S31–68

MacArthur C, Glazener CMA, Wilson PD, Herbison GP, Gee H, Lang GD, Lancashire R (2001) Obstetric practice and faecal incontinence three months after delivery. *Br J Obstet Gynaecol* **108**: 678–83

Mayerhofer K, Bodner-Adler B, Bodner K, Rabl M, Kaider A, Wagenbichler P, Armin Joura E, Husslein P (2002) Traditional care of the perineum during birth: A prospective, randomized study of 1,076 women. *J Reprod Med* **47**: 477–82

Martin S, Labrecque M, Marcoux S, Berube S, Lemiex F, Pinault JJ (2001) The association between perineal trauma and spontaneous perineal tears. *J Fam Pract* **50**: 333–7

McCandlish R, Bowler U, Van Asten H, Berridge G, Winter C, Sames L *et al* (1998) A randomised controlled trial of care of the perineum during second stage of normal labour. *Br J Obstet Gynaecol* **105**: 1262–72

Murphy PA, Feinland JB (1998) Perineal outcomes in a home birth setting. *Birth* **25**: 226–33

Payne TN, Carey JC, Rayburn WF (1999) Prior third- or fourth-degree perineal tears and recurrence risks. *Int J Gynecol Obstet* **64**: 55–7

Peleg D, Kennedy CM, Merrill D, Zlatnik FJ (1999) Risk of repetition of severe perineal laceration. *Obstet Gynecol* **93**: 1021–24

Pirhonen JP, Grenman SE, Haadem K, Gudmundsson S, Lindqvist P, Sihola S *et al* (1998) Frequency of anal sphincter rupture at delivery in Sweden and Finland — result of difference in manual help to the baby's head. *Acta Obstet Gynecol Scand* **77**: 974–7

Poen AC, Felt-Bersma RJF, Dekker GA, Deville W, Cuesta MA, Meuwissen SGM (1997) Third-degree obstetric perineal tear: Risk factors and the preventative role of mediolateral episiotomy. *Br J Obstet Gynaecol* **104**: 563–6

RCOG Audit Committee (1993) *Effective procedures in obstetrics suitable for audit.* RCOG Medical Audit Unit, Manchester

Renfrew MJ, Hannah W, Albers L, Floyd E (1998) Practices that minimize trauma to the genital tract in childbirth: A systematic review of the literature. *Birth* **25**: 143–60

Robinson CA, Macones GA, Roth WN, Morgan MA (1996) Does station of the fetal head at epidural placement affect the position of the fetal vertex at delivery? *Am J Obstet Gynecol* **175**: 991–4

Robinson JN, Norwitz ER, Cohen AP, Mcelrath TF, Lieberman ES (1999) Epidural analgesia and third- or fourth-degree lacerations in nulliparas. *Obstet Gynecol* **94**: 259–62

Rockner G, Olund A (1991) The use of episiotomy in primipara in Sweden: a descriptive study with particular focus on two hospitals. *Acta Obstet Gynecol Scand* **70**: 325–30

Royal College of Obstetricians and Gynaecologists (2000) *Methods and materials used in perineal tears.* RCOG Guideline No. 23. RCOG Press, London

Sleep J, Grant A, Garcia J, Elbourne D, Spencer J, Chalmers I (1984) West Berkshire perineal management trial. *Br Med J* **280**: 587–690

Shipman MK, Boniface DR, Tefft ME, McGlohry FM (1997) Antenatal perineal massage and susequent perineal outcomes: a randomised controlled trial. *Br J Obstet Gynaecol* **104**: 787–91

Shiono P, Klebanoff MA, Carey JC (1990) Midline episiotomies: More harm than good? *Obstet Gynecol* **75**: 765–70

Stamp G, Kruzins G, Crowther C (2001) Perineal massage in labour and prevention of perineal trauma: randomised controlled trial. *Br Med J* **322**: 1277–80

Sultan AH, Kamm MA, Hudson CN, Thomas JM, Bartram CI (1993) Anal sphincter disruption during vaginal delivery. *N Engl J Med* **329**: 1905–11

Sultan AH, Kamm MA, Hudson CN (1994a) Pudendal nerve damage during labour: prospective study before and after childbirth. *Br J Obstet Gynaecol* **101**: 22–8

Sultan AH, Kamm MA, Hudson CN, Bartram CI (1994b) Third degree obstetric anal sphincter tears: risk factors and outcome of primary repair. *Br Med J* **308**: 887–91

Sultan AH, Stanton SL (1996) Preserving the pelvic floor and perineum during childbirth — elective caesarean section? *Br J Obstet Gynaecol* **103**: 731–4

Sultan AH (1997) Anal incontinence after childbirth. *Curr Opin Obstet Gynecol* **9**: 320–4

Sultan AH, Johanson RB, Carter JE (1998) Occult anal sphincter trauma following randomized forceps and vacuum delivery. *Int J Gynecol Obstet* **61**: 113–9

Sultan AH, Monga AK, Kumar D, Stanton SL (1999) Primary repair of obstetric anal sphincter rupture using the overlap technique. *Br J Obstet Gynaecol* **106**: 318–23

Sultan AH, Thakar R (2002) Lower genital tract and anal sphincter trauma. *Best Pract & Res – Clin Obstet Gynaecol* **16**: 99–116

Thacker SB, Banta DH (1983) Benefits and risks of episiotomy: An interpretative review of the English language literature, 1860–1980. *Obstet Gynecol Surv* **38**: 322–38

Thakar R, Sultan AH, Fernando R, Monga A, Stanton S (2001) Can workshops on obstetric anal sphincter rupture change practice? Int Urogynecol J 12:S5.

Thakar R, Sultan AH (2003) Management of obstetric anal sphincter injuries. *The Obstetrician and Gynaecologist* **5**: 72–8

Woolley RJ (1995) Benefits and risks of episiotomy: a review of the English-Language Literature since 1980. Part 1 and II. *Obstet Gynaecol Surv* **50**: 806–35

# 8

## Postpartum management of the perineum

*Debra Bick*

### Introduction

Perineal morbidity is commonly experienced after childbirth, with one symptom in particular, perineal pain, frequently reported as a short and longer-term symptom (Glazener *et al*, 1995, Brown and Lumley, 1998). Pain can arise from a spontaneous tear of the perineal skin or muscle, from an episiotomy or bruising or oedema of the perineal tissues, which may occur even if the perineum is intact. If there is disruption to the perineal tissues, either spontaneously occurring, or following surgical incision, immediate management more often than not is related to the classification of trauma and the type of suturing and suturing material used to repair the trauma if required; however, following discharge from the delivery area, management is unlikely to be planned accordingly. Despite pain being experienced by hundreds of thousands of women who give birth each year in the UK, and many more worldwide (Albers *et al*, 1999; Maduma-Butshe *et al*, 1998), identification and management of perineal morbidity, including pain, dyspareunia, wound infection and haematoma has not been a high priority. The postnatal management of more severe perineal trauma, third and fourth degree tears, has also been relatively neglected.

### Postnatal care

The lack of appropriately planned and implemented postnatal care of the perineum is salutary, given the implications trauma may have for other aspects of maternal health and well-being, for example, a woman's ability to care for her baby and her relationship with her partner. As with many other areas of maternal health, women may not report symptoms of perineal pain and health professionals may not routinely ask about them. Studies of long-term maternal morbidity undertaken in several countries, have reported that for some women perineal pain persists well beyond the postnatal period (Glazener, 1997; Brown and Lumley, 1998). This chapter describes the evidence on postnatal perineal management, including short and longer-term assessment and management of pain, wound infection, dyspareunia and sexual health problems, third and fourth degree tears and haematoma. Other aspects of care which are not addressed should also be noted, for example, ensuring that excessive blood loss from the site of perineal trauma is monitored and managed appropriately.

# Perineal pain

Information on the extent and severity of perineal pain experienced following childbirth has, in the main, been obtained from studies which have included experience of pain as an outcome following implementation of a particular intervention, for example, comparison of different perineal suturing methods and materials (Kettle *et al*, 2002), following a particular mode of delivery or among different parity groups. Many of the factors studied are highly interrelated, and studies need to have undertaken appropriate multivariate analysis in order to report on the independent effects of each (Bick *et al*, 2002). No studies have evaluated the use of a tool specifically designed to measure postnatal perineal pain or capture differences in pain severity between degree of trauma, sutured and non-sutured trauma, bruising or oedema of the perineal tissues. Tools have been developed to assess levels of bruising and oedema, an example of this being the visual tool developed by Steen and Cooper (1997), which comprised life-size photographs representing degrees of severity as none, mild, moderate and severe in these outcomes. The REEDA (redness, oedema, ecchymosis, discharge and approximation) tool (Davidson, 1974) measures the degree of trauma sustained by an individual woman; however, in common with other tools, it has mainly been used to assess outcomes following a particular intervention as part of a research study, rather than inform care in day-to-day practice. A tool which has been specifically designed to measure the extent of perineal trauma in day-to-day practice has recently been validated (the Peri-Rule™, Metcalfe *et al*, 2002), and further work is being undertaken to audit impact and use (see *Chapter 6*).

Intervention studies have assessed women's experiences of perineal pain either using tools developed to measure pain across general population groups, for example visual analogue scales and numerical rating scales, or have included terms to describe severity or impact of pain on women's daily activities (Sleep, 1991). Often, several different measurements have been included in a study, data from which have been collected from self-complete or researcher administered tools.

In addition to different pain assessment measures being used, duration of time to assessment of perineal pain following the birth also differs between studies, thus making study comparisons difficult. Given the potential consequences of perineal pain for women's physical and psychological well-being, the need for effective postpartum management is imperative.

## Oral and rectal analgesics

Paracetamol is one of the most commonly used analgesics to relieve mild postnatal perineal pain (Sleep and Grant, 1988). Despite this being a readily accessible source of analgesia it may not provide an acceptable or sustainable level of pain relief for many women, and stronger analgesia may have to be considered. One major concern when considering the stronger analgesia of choice, which could include opioid or non-opioid analgesics or combinations of both, is the possibility of side-effects, particularly if women are breastfeeding.

The effectiveness of analgesic rectal suppositories for perineal pain was considered in a recent Cochrane review (Heydayati *et al*, 2004a). Rectal analgesia may be used in circumstances where oral administration is inappropriate, for example, if a woman is experiencing nausea and vomiting. One of the main advantages of rectal analgesia is that around half of the drug absorbed in the rectum will by-pass the liver and not be metabolised (Heydayati *et al*, 2004a). Studies that have assessed the use of rectal analgesia for other sources of pain, for example, following general surgery, have found it significantly reduced pain levels.

The systematic review undertaken by Heydayati *et al* (2004a) evaluated the available evidence from randomised controlled trials that assessed pain relief, maternal satisfaction and costs of using rectal analgesia for perineal pain. The reviewers identified three trials of pain relief following episiotomy or perineal tear which met review inclusion criteria, with a total of 249 women. Women who received NSAIDS suppositories compared with placebo were less likely to experience pain at or close to twenty-four hours following the delivery (RR 0.37, 95% confidence level 0.10 to 1.38). Women were also less likely to require additional analgesia in the first twenty-four hours of the birth compared with placebo (RR 0.31, 95% CI 0.17 to 0.54), an effect which was still in evidence at forty-eight hours post delivery (RR 0.63, 95% CI 0.45 to 0.89). The reviewers found no information on pain levels after three days of the birth, or effect on other outcomes, including timing of resumption of intercourse and problems experienced, or impact on maternal-infant bonding. Although rectal administration may provide more effective pain relief in the short-term, acceptability of this route of administration to postnatal women would have to be considered.

## Therapeutic ultrasound

Therapeutic ultrasound using frequencies up to 3MHz have been used in general population groups to promote healing of soft tissue injuries and fractures, with studies showing some benefit in rate of wound and bone healing. It is an application widely used by physiotherapists to heal sports-related injuries.

Amongst postnatal women, use of ultrasound to relieve pain is not a primary indication (Hay-Smith, 2004), although it has been proposed that pain is decreased due to acceleration of resolution of the inflammatory process and reduction of haematoma and oedema. Hay-Smith (2004) undertook a Cochrane review to examine the existing evidence from RCTs for the treatment of acute and/or persistent postpartum perineal pain and dyspareunia, using therapeutic ultrasound. Four trials of variable quality were identified which fulfilled review inclusion criteria, with a total of 659 women. Based on two placebo controlled trials, women treated with ultrasound for acute perineal pain were more likely to report an improvement in pain following treatment. One trial which compared pulsed electromagnetic energy with ultrasound for acute perineal pain found women treated with ultrasound were more likely to have bruising at ten days, but were less likely to have experienced perineal pain at this time. The fourth included trial, which compared outcomes among women treated with ultrasound for persistent perineal pain and/or dyspareunia, reported that they were less likely to report pain with sexual intercourse compared with the placebo group (OR 0.31, 95% CI 0.11 to 0.84). None of the other outcomes the trials assessed (including main outcomes of infant care, daily activities, sexual function, self-care; or secondary outcomes including change in severity of pain, persistence of pain, complications of wound healing) reached significance, and none of the trials assessed safety of therapeutic ultrasound or if there were any long-term effects of treatment. The conclusion of the review was that there is currently insufficient evidence to enable conclusions to be made about the benefits of therapeutic ultrasound to manage perineal injury, and further evidence from large, high quality RCTs was required.

## Local anaesthetics and non-pharmacological preparations

Topical applications to relieve pain can include use of local anaesthetics and non-pharmacological applications. Some may be more commonly used than others (for example, icepacks) to relieve postpartum perineal pain, particularly if they are readily available and can be administered by the woman herself. Examples of local anaesthetics which can be applied directly to the site of perineal injury, include lidocaine which can be administered as a spray, gel or cream, and Epifoam, an anti-inflammatory steroid-based foam. Non-pharmacological preparations include hot or cool pads, icepacks, and bathing.

Epifoam is not a widely used treatment and results of studies that have compared effectiveness of Epifoam with other topical applications have had conflicting results, for example, Moore and James (1989) reported that Epifoam was as effective as ice-packs with no delay in healing, whilst a small double-blinded RCT undertaken by Greer and Cameron (1984) found an association with Epifoam treatment and wound breakdown. An RCT undertaken by Steen *et al* (2000) compared the effectiveness of a specifically developed cooling device (maternity gel pad) on perineal morbidity, compared with two standard treatments used at the study site (icepacks and Epifoam). One-hundred and twenty women who had undergone an instrumental delivery were recruited from one midwifery unit in the north of England and randomised to one of three treatment groups; icepacks only (n = 38); epifoam only (n = 42); and gel pads only (n = 40). Women could continue to use other forms of pain relief if they wished to do so, including oral analgesia and bathing, and apply the treatments they were allocated to as required.

Main study outcomes were levels of oedema, bruising and self-assessed pain as measured using specifically developed scales at different time points during the postnatal period. These included the visual evaluating tool described earlier (Steen and Cooper, 1997) which was used by midwife assessors who were blind to treatment allocation to ascertain levels of perineal oedema and bruising at ≤4 hours, 24 hours and 48 hours, and a 10-point VAS to capture data on self-assessed pain at ≤4, 24 and 48 hours. Pain at five days after suturing was also captured using the VAS, which were administered by community midwives. Women's opinions on the effectiveness of the treatment they received was rated using a 5-point scale of poor, fair, good, very good and excellent, data on which were also collected by the community midwives at five days.

The study found that the majority of women in each group had signs of perineal oedema within four hours of their delivery, but no treatment effect was found either within four hours or at twenty-four hours. There was a significant difference in the proportion of women who had oedema at forty-eight hours, with those in the gel-pad group having less oedema. Women in the gel pad group who initially reported moderate or severe pain had a significant decrease in reported pain at forty-eight hours. There was a significant increase in the proportion of women with some bruising across all three groups from time of initial assessment up to forty-eight hours after delivery, but this was significantly less in the gel-pad group who initially had no bruising. There was no difference in treatment effect across the groups at other initial levels of severity of oedema, bruising or pain at twenty-four and forty-eight hours or pain levels at five days. Women allocated to the maternity gel-pad group were more likely to rate their treatment as effective. The researchers concluded that the gel-pads were more effective at relieving pain compared with standard treatment regimens, and more highly rated by the women who used them. As treatments were only administered whilst women were on the postnatal ward, effectiveness in the community is difficult to predict, but given the potential duration of perineal pain (Glazener, 1997), further work should be undertaken.

Icepacks have been commonly used to reduce inflammation of acute soft tissue injury, and are reported to be the most commonly used form of local treatment for perineal pain (Greenshields and Hulme, 1993). There does not appear to be a standard icepack used in postnatal care, but numerous and locally made applications (often prepared by staff on the postnatal ward) include the fingers of latex gloves and crushed ice 'sandwiched' between layers of gauze. There have been some concerns about side-effects of the use of ice on soft tissue, including vaso-constriction (Sleep, 1990), although evidence to support this is not available. Another concern is that icepacks cannot be moulded to the shape of the perineum. Given the results of the study by Steen *et al* (2000), maternity gel-pads would appear to be a more satisfactory and effective way to relieve pain by cooling.

The effectiveness of local anaesthetics will depend on the duration of pain relief they provide and strength and frequency of application (Heydayati *et al*, 2004b). Local anaesthetics have been found to be effective when used on wounds in general population studies, including pain associated with venous leg ulcers, which was the subject of a recent Cochrane review (Briggs *et al*, 2004).

A small, double blind randomised controlled trial was undertaken by researchers at a hospital in Texas to assess the efficacy of lidocaine ointment to treat pain following a vaginal delivery where the women had sustained an episiotomy or perineal laceration (Minassian *et al*, 2002). Two hundred women were randomised to receive either lidocaine (n = 108) or placebo (n = 92), with use of pain relief assessed by the amount of ointment used (by comparing the weight of the container), frequency of use of oral analgesia and completion of a pain questionnaire, which included visual and linear analogue scales. The primary outcome measure was the amount of pain relief obtained from using the ointment in the first two days post delivery.

The trial groups were similar with regard to age, parity and gestation at delivery, although there was a higher proportion of Caucasian women in the lidocaine group, a difference which was not statistically significant. There were no significant differences in amount of ointment or other forms of pain relief used on the first and second day post delivery between the groups, although a higher proportion of women randomised to the lidocaine group used other pain relief, and no difference in levels of pain or satisfaction with pain relief. Women who had sustained an episiotomy (38/37% in the intervention cf 37/44% in the placebo group) used more oral analgesia than those who had a laceration, whilst those with minor (first or second degree laceration or episiotomy) lacerations used less oral analgesia and less ointment than those who had major lacerations (third or fourth degree laceration, extended episiotomy) on the first postpartum day.

The validity and generalisability of this small study to practice outside of North America would have to be considered. No information was provided on overall recruitment rate, the authors merely stating that 'most patients agreed to participate in the study'. There was a high episiotomy rate, particularly when the majority of women had spontaneous vaginal delivery, and although this was an American study and most deliveries would have been undertaken by an obstetrician, it would still be difficult to justify the high rate given the lack of benefit to women (Eason *et al*, 2000). Consideration should also be given to potential differences in pain following performance of a median episiotomy (common practice in the USA) and a medio-lateral episiotomy (common practice in the UK). The pain questionnaire could have been completed on day one or two, and it is possible that levels of pain could have differed.

Corkhill *et al* (2001) carried out a double-blind placebo controlled trial to investigate if, topically applied, 2 per cent lignocaine gel was an effective treatment for women who had sustained a first or second degree perineal tear. One hundred and forty-nine women who delivered at one maternity unity in the north-west of England were randomised to the intervention or control group. Pain at twenty-four hours of delivery was the primary study outcome, assessed using a numerical rating scale. Secondary outcomes included pain at forty-eight hours, need for oral analgesia and maternal satisfaction. Women who used the gel had lower average pain scores, however this was only significant at forty-eight hours post-delivery, with no difference in use of oral analgesia. As this was a secondary outcome based on a small group of women (the study was not powered to detect this difference), larger studies are needed to assess the effectiveness of the gel in the immediate and longer-term postnatal period.

## Bathing

Bathing in water with salt additives has traditionally been used to relieve wound pain and promote healing. A three-arm randomised controlled trial examined the effectiveness of adding salt, a 25ml sachet of 'Savlon' or nothing to bath water each day for the first ten days after delivery (Sleep and Grant, 1988). One thousand and eight hundred women who had a vaginal delivery were randomised to one of the three groups and outcomes assessed at ten days and three months. At ten days, the prevalence of perineal pain and pattern of wound healing was similar between the groups, and at three months pain levels remained similar. Timing of resumption of intercourse and experience of dyspareunia did not differ at three months. Although bath additives did not reduce pain or dyspareunia or enhance healing, most of the women reported that bathing did provide some relief of the discomfort they were experiencing.

## Alternative therapies

The use of lavender oil, synthetic lavender oil or an inert oil added to bath water to relieve perineal pain was examined in an RCT (Dale and Cornwell, 1994). Six hundred and thirty-five women were randomised to one of the three groups and asked to add oil to their bathwater every day for ten days post delivery. A visual analogue scale was used to assess daily discomfort, but no differences in pain levels were found between the groups. Other remedies, such as arnica, are also used by women to relieve perineal pain (Greenshields and Hulme, 1993); however, further trials are required to assess the safety and benefit of alternative therapies.

## Perineal wound infection

Delay in the healing of perineal trauma could contribute to long-term experience of pain and other morbidity. In common with aspects of wound care management among the general population, there is no standard definition of postpartum perineal wound infection, limited information on onset, incidence and prevalence and no evidence of effective management or resources. As with perineal pain, data on wound infections tend to have been collated as an outcome of studies of perineal management during and immediately following delivery; for example, the use of different suturing materials (Kettle *et al*, 2002), or from large surveys of postnatal health, as reported by Cathryn Glazener in *Chapter 2*.

In Glazener's 1999 survey of 707 women who had spontaneous or assisted vaginal delivery (*Chapter 2*), 5.5% had perineal wound breakdown. One large observational study in France which included 2000 women who had their episiotomies sutured with polyglactin 910 suture material, 2% of women reported wound dehiscence at three days postpartum (Masson *et al*, 1988).

Some data on infection are also available from retrospective data analysis. Perineal wound infections have been reported following severe perineal trauma, for example fourth degree tears. Goldaber *et al* (1993) undertook a retrospective case review of women who had sustained fourth degree tears during 1989 and 1990 at a hospital in Texas, USA. Of three hundred and ninety women who sustained a fourth degree tear, twenty-one (5.4%) had postpartum perineal morbidity, seven (1.8%) of whom had wound dehiscence alone, eleven (2.8%) had infection and dehiscence and three (0.8%) had infection alone. When factors that could predict perineal morbidity were examined, women with morbidity were more likely to have experienced shoulder dystocia, metritis and postpartum pyrexia. One of the main problems with retrospective studies is that data may be incomplete, as women may not have developed infection until after hospital discharge and may have been treated at home or at another unit.

Perineal suturing methods and the type of suturing material used may have implications for risk of development of a wound infection. A recent trial of continuous versus interrupted perineal repair using standard or rapidly absorbed sutures following a normal vaginal delivery (Kettle *et al*, 2002) found when comparing suturing methods that suture removal was lower in women who had received continuous sutures. There was also less wound gaping at ten days in this group. When suturing materials were compared, rate of suture material removal was significantly lower among women whose perineal trauma had been sutured using polylgactin 910 suture material (p<0.0001), which is a more rapidly absorbed material.

In the absence of information on perineal wound breakdown, signs and symptoms of surgical wound breakdown from caesarean section and general population studies have been considered, data from which are usually based on studies of healing by primary intention (where the edges of the wound have been brought together and closed using sutures). However, unlike a general surgical wound, perineal wounds will not be protected by a dressing and some may not be sutured, where healing is referred to as taking place by 'secondary intention'. Risk factors for delayed wound healing, include; poor nutrition, anaemia, number of bacteria and host resistance, and type of surgery performed (Sharp and McLaws, 2004). A definition of degree of contamination of surgical operative site was outlined by McClaws and Caelli (2000) and published in the

*American Journal of Infection Control.* Wounds to the genital, respiratory, alimentary or urinary tract are defined as 'clean-contaminated wounds', which are operative wounds, 'in which the..... tract is entered under controlled conditions and without unusual contamination'.

The majority of studies of wound infection following caesarean section have been retrospective and subject to the same sorts of bias as described earlier, but most found that the common time of occurrence of wound infection was between four and five days after delivery (Leigh *et al*, 1990). Signs and symptoms which indicated possible wound infection included pyrexia, localised pain and erythema, excess exudate, odour and localised oedema. Signs of wound dehiscence (separation of the wound edges) should also be noted. In the absence of definition of perineal wound infection, it is likely that these are also symptoms which would indicate the presence of infection in the perineum. Prevention of infection is also an important part of postnatal care. Care to prevent perineal wound infection should include discussing with the woman the importance of good general hygiene, for example; ensuring that she is aware that sanitary pads should be changed regularly, that she uses correct hand washing techniques, the perineal area is kept clean by regular bathing or showering and that her dietary intake includes foods rich in vitamin C which promote wound healing.

Women who have sustained perineal trauma should be asked about symptoms as described above and if infection is suspected, wound swabs for culture and sensitivity should be taken in accordance with local policies. Obstetrician or GP referral (depending on where the woman is being cared for) should be made as antibiotics may be required. Some women may require re-suturing of their perineal trauma which should be undertaken as soon as possible, and consideration given to the type of suture material used; for example, standard vicryl which does not dissolve may be more appropriate than using vicryl rapide to enable the area to heal (Kettle, personal communication). A decision may be taken to leave the wound to heal by secondary intent. Further work is required to ensure that accurate data on the onset, frequency and type of perineal wound infection experienced are collected to ensure postnatal practitioners are aware of these and can identify, manage and discuss care with women.

## Dyspareunia and sexual health problems

The assessment and management of dyspareunia (pain experienced before, during or following sexual intercourse) which is more likely to be associated with perineal pain (Glazener, 1997) is also a neglected area, with few studies investigating the identification or management of this symptom and a dearth of information on onset and duration. Data that are available tend to have been obtained from observational studies and trials of different perineal management regimens (Kettle *et al*, 2002), and as is the case for perineal pain, data are usually restricted to different parity and delivery types (Bick *et al*, 2002). As well as physical factors, pain on intercourse may also be triggered by psychosocial factors (Morris and Mukhophadyay, 2003), some of which may have been present before the pregnancy. If dyspareunia has been investigated, more often than not it has been included in a questionnaire survey and women asked to respond to questions to recall when intercourse was resumed and their experiences of problems, which may be subject to recall bias.

Recent work on women's sexual health after childbirth has shown that sexual health problems are common, although few are identified by health professionals or reported by the women. Barrett *et al* (2000) undertook a cross-sectional study of all primiparous women who had delivered at one unit in London during a six-month period. Seven hundred and ninety-six women were sent a postal questionnaire which inquired about their general health, bowel and bladder function, mental health and experiences of a range of sexual health problems and sexual behaviour before and after the pregnancy. Of 484 (61%) women who responded, 32% had resumed intercourse within six weeks of the birth, and the majority of the respondents (89%) had resumed intercourse within six months. Sexual health problems, as recalled by the women, increased significantly following the birth. In the first three months, 83% had experienced sexual problems, which declined to 64% at six months although this was still higher than recall of problems before the pregnancy which were reported by 38% of the women. Dyspareunia, which was defined as pain on penetration and/or pain during intercourse or orgasm, was reported by 62% of women at some time during three months of giving birth, half of whom still experienced this at six months. Dyspareunia in the first three months of the birth was significantly associated with a vaginal delivery and previous experience of dyspareunia. However, at six months, only previous experience of dyspareunia was significant. Although the response rate to this study was 61%, suggesting that prevalence of symptoms is under reported, the fact that only 15% of women had discussed their problems with a health professional highlights the high level of unmet need in relation to sexual well-being.

Risk factors for sexual health problems experienced after childbirth have been identified from obstetric factors. These are parity, mode of delivery and perineal trauma. Some of these factors could be minimised, as described in *Chapter 7* of this book, however others cannot be controlled for, highlighting the importance of care to reduce the experience of postnatal morbidity. Women should be asked if they have resumed sexual intercourse, and if they have, if they experienced any pain or discomfort. As research has shown that many women will have resumed intercourse within the first six to eight weeks postpartum (Klein *et al*, 1994; Glazener 1997), it is important that the midwife or other health professional includes sexual well-being as part of a woman's overall assessment sooner rather than later in the postnatal period. There is a dearth of information with regard to management of postpartum dyspareunia, with trials of routine versus intensive pelvic floor exercises finding no difference in prevalence of dyspareunia at three months postpartum (Sleep and Grant, 1987), a similar finding to the RCT of bath additives described earlier (Sleep and Grant, 1988).

Greenshields and Hulme (1993) in a large survey of members of the National Childbirth Trust, reported that some women rubbed oils or gels on their perineums or used vaginal lubrication to relieve soreness on penetration, or used relaxation techniques during intercourse. Women who are breastfeeding may find this information beneficial, as it was been shown in the study by Barrett *et al* (2000), referred to earlier, that they may be more likely to experience vaginal dryness. It is also important to ensure that women who are depressed or at risk of developing depression are identified and managed appropriately, as this could have implications for their sexual health. Morof *et al* (2003) undertook further analysis of women who participated in the study by Barrett *et al* (2000), and asked them to complete the Edinburgh Postnatal Depression Scale (EPDS) in addition to answering questions on their sexual health. Of the 484 original respondents, 468 (97%) completed the EPDS, fifty-seven (12%) of whom had a score of thirteen or more (who were classed as depressed). Women who were depressed were significantly less likely to have resumed intercourse by six months postpartum than women who were not depressed (13/23.2% cf 40/9.8%). The pattern of sexual problems did not differ between depressed and non-depressed women, although the median number of specific sexual problems experienced by depressed women was two compared with one in non-depressed women (p<0.009).

As the researchers point out, causality cannot be ascertained, however women who are depressed may have a more negative view of their bodies and health, which could be triggers for symptoms of depression. Interestingly, when perineal trauma was studied for possible association with depression, no relationship was found. These researchers called for more research to be undertaken on the partner's feelings and risk for postnatal depression and to determine the relationship between sexual satisfaction, dyspareunia and postnatal depression. They also emphasise that sexual health problems should not be viewed as symptoms only triggered by adverse psychological well-being, given the high proportion of problems experienced by depressed and non-depressed women.

## Third and fourth degree tears

Management of a woman's perineum following immediate delivery care, whether in hospital or at home, is rarely based on the level of trauma sustained. Exceptions to this may include (but not always) management of third or fourth degree tears, which documented cases suggest are experienced by around 4% of women (Sultan *et al*, 1994) and are associated with an increased risk of developing faecal incontinence, in addition to pain, dyspareunia and infection (Wood *et al*, 1998; Fenner *et al*, 2003; Fernando *et al*, 2004). One major concern in relation to this type of delivery injury is whether midwives and obstetricians are able correctly to identify and repair damage to the anal sphincter and epithelium, as described in *Chapter 7* and it is likely that incidence is under-reported. This situation may be compounded by a lack of agreement in the description of the extent of trauma involving the anal sphincter (Fernando *et al*, 2004). Risk factors for obstetric anal sphincter injury have been identified as instrumental delivery, midline episiotomy, infant birth weight and OP position at delivery.

There is little information to guide postpartum care of women who sustain this type of perineal trauma. Expert opinion is that prophylactic laxatives (lactulose or fybogel) should be prescribed to prevent constipation and women should not be discharged until they have had their bowels opened (Sultan, 1999). Dietary advice may also be of benefit. Antibiotics should also be prescribed to prevent infection, although the benefit of these regimens is uncertain (Bick *et al*, 2002). The effectiveness of a behavioural technique, biofeedback, has been assessed to manage women who are symptomatic, although studies to date have been small. Fynes *et al* (1999) randomly assigned thirty-six women who developed faecal incontinence after an anal sphincter tear and three after a traumatic vaginal delivery to receive sensory (which uses pelvic floor muscle exercises together with sensory feedback from a perinometer, n = 19) or augmented biofeedback (which includes electrical stimulation of the anal sphincter with audiovisual electromyography feedback, n = 20). Continence scores had improved in both groups after twelve weeks of treatment, but results were better for women in the augmented biofeedback group. Further studies involving larger groups of women are required.

Women may require surgery to repair the anal sphincter, although the long-term effectiveness of type of repair (end to end or overlap) is unknown, and a Cochrane review of methods of repair for obstetric anal sphincter injury is being developed (Fernando *et al*, 2004). Other areas that require evaluation include type of suturing material used, the most appropriate person to perform the repair and mode of delivery for a future pregnancy. Some obstetric units have established postnatal perineal clinics for women who have sustained third or fourth degree tears and/or developed faecal incontinence or have other symptoms including perineal pain, where symptoms can be identified, investigated and managed. A recent audit of the characteristics of 399 women who attended a dedicated perineal clinic at a maternity unit in Dublin during 1998–1999 demonstrated the value of this service for those who had sustained severe perineal trauma (Fitzpatrick *et al*, 2002), however the extent of provision of clinics is unknown.

## Haematoma

A haematoma may occur in the vulval, vaginal or sub-peritoneal areas either immediately following delivery or in the days or weeks following the birth. They occur infrequently, with an incidence of between 1 in 500 and 1 in 900 pregnancies (Ridgway, 1995; Villella *et al*, 2001) and if a haematoma does develop, it can be extremely painful if blood loss is large, potentially life-threatening.

Care should be taken when examining the perineum in the immediate and longer-term postnatal period to ensure that the whole perineal area is observed, as the site of a haematoma may be obscured or missed if a detailed examination is not undertaken. Prompt identification and management are essential as delay could lead to significant blood loss. Incision and drainage, followed by suturing and packing of the site may have to be undertaken to relieve symptoms as first line management (Propst and Thorp, 1998). Two case reports of angiographic embolisation which were required when first line management failed to achieve haemostasis were reported as successful procedures, with neither woman showing evidence of further haematoma formation at six weeks postpartum (Villella *et al*, 2001).

## The international perspective

Appropriate postnatal management of the perineum should be an integral component of care wherever a woman has given birth. This chapter has summarised evidence from a range of studies, most of which were undertaken in the developed world where some form of postnatal follow-up will be provided. Although the care provider may have differed from country to country, six to eights weeks was generally considered as the duration of the postnatal period. What is clear is that the majority of women across the globe who have a vaginal delivery will experience some form of perineal morbidity, and in many countries practices that have no benefit or, indeed, which may be harmful, continue to be implemented. Differences in the provision of care available should not deflect from the need to ensure that evidence of best practice to reduce immediate and longer-term morbidity is implemented, which includes care during the antepartum, intrapartum as well as postpartum period. More urgent and a greater challenge still is the need to implement evidence into practice for women and their babies at greatest risk of morbidity and mortality.

# References

Albers L, Garcia J, Renfrew M, McCandlish R, Elbourne D (1999) Distribution of genital tract trauma in childbirth and related postnatal pain. *Birth* **26**: 11–15

Barrett G, Pendry E, Peacock J *et al* (2000) Women's sexual problems after childbirth. *Br J Obstet Gynaecol* **107**(2): 186–95

Bick D, MacArthur C, Knowles H, Winter H (2002) *Postnatal Care. Evidence and Guidelines for Management*. Churchill Livingstone, Edinburgh

Briggs M, Nelson EA (2004) Topical agents or dressings for pain in venous leg ulcers (Cochrane Review). In: The Cochrane Library, Issue 1. John Wiley and Sons, Ltd, Chichester

Brown S, Lumley J (1998) Maternal health after childbirth: results of an Australian based survey. *Br J Obstet Gynaecol* **105**: 156–61

Corkhill A, Lavender T, Walkinshaw SA, Alfirevic Z (2001). Reducing postnatal pain from perineal tears by using lignocaine gel: a double-blind randomized trial. *Birth* **28**(1): 22–7

Dale A, Cornwall S (1994) The role of lavender oil in relieving perineal discomfort following childbirth: a blind randomized controlled trial. *J Adv Nurs* **19**(1): 89–96

Davidson N (1974) REEDA: evaluating postpartum healing. *J Nurse Midwifery* **19**: 6–9

Eason E, Labreque M, Wells G, Feldman P (2000) Preventing perineal trauma during childbirth: a systematic review. *Obstet Gynecol* **95**(3): 464–71

Fenner DE, Genberg B, Brahma P, Marek L, DeLancy JO (2003) Fecal and urinary incontinence after vaginal delivery with anal sphincter disruption in an obstetrics unit in the United States. *Am J Obstet Gynecol* **189**: 1543–50

Fernando R, Johanson R, Kettle C, Sultan A, Radley S (2004) Methods of repair for obstetric anal sphincter injury (Protocol for a Cochrane Review). In: The Cochrane Library, Issue 1. John Wiley and Sons Ltd, Chichester

Fitzpatrick M, Cassidy M, Ronan O'Connell, O'Herlihy (2002) Experience with an obstetric perineal clinic. *Europ J Obstet Gynecol* **100**: 199–203

Fynes MM, Donnelley V, Cassidy M *et al* (1999) A prospective, randomized study comparing the effect of augmented biofeedback with sensory biofeedback alone on fecal incontinence after obstetric trauma. *Dis Colon Rectum* **42**(6): 753–61

Glazener CMA, Abdalla A, Stroud P *et al* (1995) Postnatal maternal morbidity: extent, causes, prevention and treatment. *Br J Obstet Gynaecol* **102**: 282–87

Glazener CMA (1997) Sexual function after childbirth: women's experiences, persistent morbidity and lack of professional recognition. *Br J Obstet Gynaecol* **104**: 330–35

Goldaber KG, Wendel PJ, McIntire DD, Wendel GD Jr (1993) Postpartum perineal morbidity after fourth-degree perineal repair. *Am J Obstet Gynecol* **168**(2): 489–93

Greenshields W, Hulme H (1993) *The Perineum in Childbirth. A Survey of Women's Experiences and Midwifery Practices*.The National Childbirth Trust, London

Greer IA, Cameron AD (1984) Topical pramoxine and hydrocortisone foam versus placebo in relief of post-partum episiotomy symptoms and wound healing. *Scot Med J* **29**: 104–6

Hay-Smith EJC (2004) Therapeutic ultrasound for postpartum perineal pain and dyspareunia (Cochrane Review). In: The Cochrane Library, Issue 1. John Wiley and Sons Ltd, Chichester

Hedayati H, Parsons J, Crowther CA (2004a) Rectal analgesia for pain from perineal trauma following childbirth (Cochrane Review). In: The Cochrane Library, Issue 1. John Wiley and Sons Ltd, Chichester

Hedayati H, Parsons J, Crowther CA (2004b) Topically applied anaesthetics for treatment of perineal pain after childbirth (Protocol for a Cochrane Review). In: The Cochrane Library, Issue 1. John Wiley and Sons Ltd, Chichester

Kamm MA (1998) Faecal incontinence. *Br Med J* **316**: 528–32

Kettle C, Hills RK, Jones P, Darby L, Gray, Johanson R (2002) Continuous versus interrupted perineal repair with standard or rapidly absorbed sutures after spontaneous vaginal birth: a randomised controlled trial. *Lancet* **359**: 2217–23

Klein MC, Gauthier RJ, Robbins JM *et al* (1994) Relationship of episiotomy to perineal trauma and morbidity, sexual dysfunction and pelvic floor relaxation. *Am J Obstet Gynecol* **171**(3): 591–98

Leigh DA, Emmanuel FXS, Sedgwick J *et al* (1990) Post-operative urinary tract infection and wound infection in women undergoing caesarean section: a comparison of two study periods in 1985 and 1987. *J Hosp Infect* **15**: 107–16

Maduma-Butshe A, Dyall A, Garner P (1998) Routine episiotomy in developing countries. *Br Med J* **316**: 1179–80

McLaws ML, Caelli M (2000) Pilot testing standardized surveillance: Hospital Infection Standardised Surveillance (HISS). *Am J Infect Control* **28**(6): 401–5

Masson F, Bilweis J, Di Lucca D, Trentsaux G, Wrube H (1988) Interest ina new suture material for 2000 episiotomy repairs: Polyglactin 410. *Clinique Gynécologique et Obstétricale*: 19–21

Metcalfe A, Tohill S, Williams A, Haldon V, Brown L, Henry L (2002) A pragmatic tool for the measurement of perineal tears. *Br J Midwif* **10**(7): 412–17

Minassian VA, Allahyar J, Prien SD, Timmons RL, Stumbo K (2002) Randomized Trial of Lidocaine Ointment Versus Placebo for the Treatment of Postpartum Perineal Pain. *Obstet Gynecol* **100**: 1239–43

Moore W, James DK (1989) A random trial of three topical analgesic agents in the treatment of episiotomy pain following instrumental vaginal delivery. *J Obstet Gynaecol* **10**: 35–9

Morof D, Barrett G, Peacock J, Victor CR, Manyonda I (2003) Postnatal depression and sexual health after childbirth. *Am J Obstet Gynecol* **102**(6): 1318–25

Morris E, Mukhophadyay S (2003) Dyspareunia in gynaecological practice. *Curr Obstet Gynaecol* **13**: 232–8

Propst AM, Thorp JM Jr (1998) Traumatic vulvar hematomas: conservative versus surgical management. *Southern Med J* **91**(2): 144–6

Ridgway L (1995) Puerperal emergency. Vaginal and vulvar haematomas. *Obstet Gynecol Clin N Am* **22**(2): 275–82

Sleep J, Grant A (1987) Pelvic floor exercises in postnatal care — the report of a randomised controlled trial to compare an intensive exercise regimen with the programme in current use. *Midwifery* **3**: 158–64

Sleep J, Grant A (1988) Relief of perineal pain following childbirth: a survey of midwifery practice. *Midwifery* **4**: 118–22

Sleep J (1990) Postnatal perineal care. In: Alexander J, Levy V, Roch S, eds. *Postnatal Care: a research based approach*. Macmillan, London

Sleep J (1991) Perineal Care, a series of 5 randomized controlled trials. In: Robinson S, Thomson A, eds. *Midwives Research and Childbirth*. Chapman Hall, London: 200

Sharp CA, McLaws M (2004) Wound dressings for surgical sites (Protocol for a Cochrane Review). In: The Cochrane Library, Issue 1. John Wiley and Sons Ltd, Chichester

Steen M, Cooper K, Marchant P, Griffiths-Jones, Walker J (2000) A randomised controlled trial to compare the effectiveness of icepacks and Epifoam with cooling maternity gel pads at alleviating postnatal perineal trauma. *Midwifery* **16**: 48–55

Steen M, Cooper K (1997) A tool for assessing perineal trauma. *J Wound Care* **6**(9): 432–6

Sultan AH, Kamm MA, Hudson CN, Bartram CI (1994) Third degree obstetric anal sphincter tears: risk factors and outcome of primary repair. *Br Med J* **308**: 887–91

Sultan AH (1999) Obstetrical perineal injury and anal incontinence. *Clinical Risk* **5**: 193–6

Villella J, Garry D, Levine G, Glanz S, Figueroa R, Maulik D (2001) Postpartum angiographic embolization for vulvovaginal hematoma. A report of two cases. *J Reprod Med* **46**(1): 65–7

Wood J, Amos L, Rieger N (1998) Third degree anal sphincter tears: risk factors and outcome. *Aust NZ J Obstet Gynaecol* **38**: 414–17

# Concluding remarks

*Christine Henderson and Debra Bick*

Making pregnancy and childbirth safer continues to be a worldwide activity of the greatest importance. Reducing the number of women dying in childbirth by three-quarters by 2015 is one of the key goals of the Millennium Declaration of the United Nations.

Every minute, a woman dies from complications related to pregnancy and childbirth — that means 1600 deaths every day — more than half a million deaths every year worldwide. Ninety-nine per cent of these deaths occur in the developing world. In addition, for every woman who dies in childbirth, around fifteen to thirty more suffer injury, infection, disease, infertility, pelvic pain, incontinence or obstetric fistula — approximately ten million women each year. For postnatal women one of the commonest morbidities is a painful perineum. This can have a profound effect on the most basic daily activities for women and can destroy families.

This book has endeavoured to raise issues surrounding women's health worldwide, to give an international view and also to focus specifically on the perineum because, when damaged, it can have such a devastating effect on women and their families. Moreover, the contributors to this book have examined the evidence and highlighted ways that can help to prevent and/or reduce the damage sustained.

Perineal trauma is an international problem in developed and developing world countries alike. All countries need to develop strategies that ensure women receive care during their pregnancy, labour and postnatal period which is underpinned by evidence of benefit in the shorter and longer-term. In some countries, some practices may be more difficult than others to implement due to resource implications, but this should not discourage all relevant carers to work together to improve care and implement measures to prevent and limit the impact of perineal morbidity that are within their control.

Contributors to this book have highlighted the following areas that could improve practice, thus preventing and reducing the suffering that some women experience when the perineum is damaged.

There needs to be:

- Adequate training in the recognition of the extent of perineal trauma of those attending women in childbirth.
- Improved knowledge of the structures involved when tears or incisions are made to the perineum during childbirth.
- Greater understanding of how wounds heal.
- Access to evidence for those involved in childbirth.
- Early recognition and appropriate repair of trauma.
- Appropriate use of the correct materials to repair damage.
- Experienced personnel to suture damaged tissue.

- ⌘ Short- and long-term follow-up to include dedicated perineal clinics consisting of midwives, obstetricians and ano-rectal surgeons.
- ⌘ Standard recording of the level of trauma sustained at delivery; for example, using the Peri-Rule™ and establishing a national database.
- ⌘ Regular audit and feedback as part of clinical practice.
- ⌘ Development of a prescribing policy.

There is a dearth of evidence of the long-term benefit of current management. Research in this area of practice should include:

- ⌘ Dissemination and implementation strategies to sustain best practice.
- ⌘ Prospective cohort studies of risk factors, outcome and impact of morbidity.
- ⌘ Rigorously conducted and evaluated randomised controlled trials of clinical and cost-effective postnatal management options.
- ⌘ Robust evaluation of the impact of changes in practice, for example, suturing versus non-suturing.

The symptoms that women experience from perineal trauma are widespread and persistent. The problem of identifying the true global incidence of perineal trauma is due to the inconsistency in classification of trauma and under reporting of labour outcomes. Women suffer in silence but it can affect their baby, family and community with economic repercussions. Prevention and minimisation of trauma should be an international priority.

# Index